SPEECH AFTER LARYNGECTOMY

SPEECH AFTER LARYNGECTOMY

A Comparative Study of the Breathing and Speech Coordinations of Laryngectomized and Normal Subjects, and the Relationships Between the Breathing and Speech Coordinations and Articulatory Errors of Laryngectomized Subjects to their Speech Intelligibility

Louis M. Di Carlo
Walter W. Amster
Gilbert R. Herer
Syracuse University

SYRACUSE UNIVERSITY PRESS – 1955

SYRACUSE UNIVERSITY
SPECIAL EDUCATION AND REHABILITATION
MONOGRAPH SERIES I
WILLIAM M. CRUICKSHANK, *editor*

This study was supported in part by control project grant No. CS-9271 from the National Cancer Institute, National Institute of Health, Public Health Service.

Dedicated to

DR. IRL H. BLAISDELL,

Surgeon, Scholar, Research Worker, whose untimely death terminated a brilliant career and took from us a great humanitarian.

FOREWORD

Surgical removal of the larynx represents only one of the factors in the rehabilitation of the laryngectomized patient. The surgeon must be willing to devote time, effort, and thought to the psychological and social problems of his patients. The ability to speak after laryngectomy becomes of crucial importance to the individual. The surgeon's responsibility therefore extends beyond the operative care stage and should provide for an adequate orientation program from the beginning. Such an orientation would involve the participation and contribution of other specialties.

This monograph presents an interesting and instructive study of speech production after laryngectomy. The authors have endeavored to understand and quantify some of the factors involved in the speech of laryngectomized persons. While previous investigators have studied speech production after laryngectomy, the authors' use of cinefluorographic techniques has helped to clarify the area and manner of production of the voice.

Their tentative conclusions based on their findings provide a rationale and framework for a systematic program of speech training after laryngectomy.

Cleveland, Ohio   JULIUS W. McCALL, M.D.

ACKNOWLEDGMENTS

The authors wish to express their indebtedness to Dr. Eric F. Gardner and Dr. George G. Thompson of the Syracuse University faculty for their careful evaluation and guidance and pertinent suggestions which contributed to the final form of the project. To Dr. Ramon L. Irwin and Dr. Joseph M. Masling, also of the Syracuse University Faculty, acknowledgment is gratefully extended for their careful reading of the manuscript.

To Dr. Clarence V. Hudgins of the Clark School for the Deaf, Northampton, Massachusetts, we express our sincere appreciation for his constructive criticism and invaluable suggestions with respect to instrumentation and measurement and also for his careful reading of the manuscript.

It is also a pleasure to acknowledge the important contributions of Dr. J. S. Watson, Dr. G. H. Ramsey and Dr. R. Graniak, of the Strong Memorial Hospital, Rochester Medical School, Rochester, New York, for their kindness in making available their cinefluoroscopic equipment; for their time and effort, which made possible the completion of the cinefluoroscopic film of the physiological and anatomical mechanism involved in speech after laryngectomy.

Appreciation is also extended to Dr. Gordon D. Hoople, Medical Director of the Gordon D. Hoople Hearing and Speech Center; Dr. David Brewer and the late Dr. Irl H. Blaisdell of Syracuse, New York, who evaluated the surgical data and the cinefluorographic film views and assisted in securing subjects for the study.

Our sincere thanks are expressed to the auditors who gave freely of their time and energies in cooperating in this project.

To Mrs. Jean M. Gilman of Syracuse, New York, credit is expressed for her painstaking efforts in proofreading, typing, and completing the manuscript in its present form.

Our deep gratitude is expressed to all individuals who served as subjects in this investigation.

While the contributions of all the individuals mentioned have aided in completion of the final form of the project, the authors alone assume responsibility for any inadequacies.

Louis M. Di Carlo
Walter W. Amster
Gilbert R. Herer

Syracuse University

CONTENTS

LIST OF FIGURES

xiii

LIST OF TABLES

CHAPTER ONE

INTRODUCTION

THE REHABILITATION OF THE LARYNGECTOMIZED IN-
dividual presents a multiplicity of problems and is recognized as a
diverse and complex process requiring a team approach including the
services of the medical, psychological, vocational and educational specialties. Psychodynamics of individual and social behavior consistent
with good mental hygiene principles must teach the laryngectomized
individual to deal with frustration adequately and prevent the precipi-
tation of psychotic episodes. Schall (48) lists some of the possible factors
that might precipitate emotional shock after laryngectomy: (1) inability
to utter a sound, (2) the changed feeling concerning breathing, (3) the
loss of the sense of smell, (4) the changed taste of food, (5) the inability
to cough.

Despite refinement in research techniques and the advancement of
early detection methods for cancer of the larynx, total excision of the
larynx is still observed in the majority of cases. Today, however, the
problem of the laryngectomized person is recognized as entailing more
than the mere excision of the larynx. McCall insists that medical treat-
ment of the laryngectomized is but one facet of the total rehabilitation
process for these individuals.

> If the surgeon is not willing to devote much time, effort and thought
> to patients who undergo this operation, to their social and psychologic
> problems and to their rehabilitation, he should not undertake their man-
> agement. . . . The laryngeal surgeon's responsibility should now extend
> beyond the operative care and should provide systematic training to insure
> a speaking voice after operation, for this is of prime importance to the
> patient. (38), p. 10.

As early as 1858 Czermak (10) conceived of the possibility of producing voice and speech by conducting the air stream issuing from the
tracheal opening into the mouth through a tube containing a reed
capable of vibrating. He also suggested the possibility of producing
speech without the use of a mechanical vibrating reed. He felt that the
slight amount of air contained in the pharyngeal or oral cavities acting
as an air column in combination with articulatory movements might
provide a means of producing speech. He came to these conclusions

1

during a study of a patient with complete laryngeal stenosis, whose breathing for respiration was carried on independently through a tracheal stoma.

In 1873 Billroth (6) performed the first laryngectomy for cancer of the larynx. Since then progress in the sciences has contributed to the refinement and elaboration of surgical techniques; better methods of early discovery and more adequate diagnosis of cancer of the larynx has established laryngectomy as an accepted life-saving procedure.

Today concomitant rehabilitation methodology both precedes and follows the operation, since the reestablishment of communication becomes paramount in the social rehabilitation of these individuals. Stoerk (60) in 1887 published one of the first reports of a patient who developed pseudo-voice following total laryngectomy for cancer. In 1908, Gutzman Sr. (20) reported a study of twenty-five laryngectomized persons whom he taught to speak intelligibly without the use of artificial larynges. These reports of intelligible speech, produced without mechanical means, stimulated the teaching of pseudo-voice and served to highlight some of the disadvantages of artificial larynges.

Seeman in 1926 indicated several disadvantages of laryngeal prostheses:

1. Artificial larynges are embarrassing to the wearer and continue to remind him of his handicap.
2. They are unreliable and would often deteriorate mechanically.
3. The voice quality produced was unnatural and monotonous.
4. Continued use of the prosthesis might cause recurrence of cancer from prolonged irritation of the tissue.

One can say today that the artificial larynx has completely lost its significance as a substitute for voice because it is possible to teach each laryngectomized person to speak loudly and distinctly and thereby to make him independent from any and every voice prosthesis. The artificial larynx belongs to the past; its application must today be regarded as a backward step which cannot be reconciled to the newest progresses of phoniatry. (51) p. 287.

Although Morrison (41), Stetson (55), and Kallen (32) later acknowledged that speech through the use of artificial larynges might be employed as a means of communication, nevertheless they concerned themselves more fully with the various types of pseudo-voice that could be produced without mechanical means.

Kallen (32) classified several types of pseudo-voice:

1. The pseudo-whisper, which involves a compression of the air in the oral cavity acting in combination with the articulatory movements of the consonant sounds for the production of speech.
2. Pharyngeal voice.

3. Esophageal voice.
4. Gastric voice.

The last three types of pseudo-voice differ primarily in the probable locations of the vicarious air chamber and pseudo-glottis.

Stetson classified two distinct types of esophageal voice. In the first type of esophageal speech:

> The subject gulps a large amount of air, retains it probably in the stomach, and speaks his phrase on one long, hasty, belching 'breath.' The air in the stomach will be subject to pressure variations from the chest. . . . In the second type of oesophageal speech the subject takes a few c.c. of air into the upper oesophagus, forces it through the pharyngo-oesophageal slit to produce his syllables. The supply of air must be very frequently renewed. (57), p. 99.

Nelson, in a training manual written primarily for the laryngectomized individual, outlines therapy procedures for two types of speech:

1. The pharyngeal speech method.
2. The esophageal speech method.

> The air that enters the mouth and nose is locked in the throat by placing the tip of the tongue against the lower rear of the front gums of the mouth. The tongue is arched so that the center of the tongue touches the roof of the mouth just as if you were making the sound KUH. By pushing the arched part of the tongue hard against the roof and forward a slight thump will be felt in the throat. When this occurs make a sound immediately before you lose the air that you have locked. (43), pp. 42-47.

The esophageal method, according to Nelson, entails a swallowing of the air and pressure on the stomach to force a belching sound from the throat. He suggests that the subject take and hold a deep breath before swallowing. Nelson, a laryngectomized person who taught himself to speak, considers the pharyngeal speech method superior, since it permits more rapid locking of the air, allowing more natural phrasing for communication purposes.

These various classifications of pseudo-voice introduce basic considerations and constructs in teaching the laryngectomized to speak, which evolve about the controversy concerning the location of, (1) the vicarious air chamber, (2) the site of the pseudo-glottis.

Because of the multitudinous classifications and consequent confusions resulting from the speculations concerning the location of the air chamber and the glottis, it would appear desirable to designate any phonated speech without artificial larynx as *speech after laryngectomy*. This terminology will be adhered to throughout this study.

Speech communication for the laryngectomized person becomes a personal and social imperative. The establishment of the communication arc in which the individual interacts with his environment becomes the primary goal of the rehabilitation process after surgery. The necessary return to their environment as efficient functioning members must occur in a minimum amount of time.

If the acquisition of speech becomes too difficult and too prolonged and if the acquired speech is not operationally efficient, the tendency toward withdrawal and compensatory behavior becomes the most likely means of adjustment since it presents the most efficient method of tension reduction.

To insure adequate adjustment, speech for the laryngectomized person should be functional and acceptable to him and to others. To understand the speech problems of the laryngectomized person a consideration of normal speech coordinations is important. Normal speech breathing coordinations have been studied extensively by Stetson (56) and by Hudgins (23).

The fundamental unit of speech is the syllable produced by the ballistic action of the chest muscles. The larger abdominal muscles support the action of the chest musculature in producing a series of syllables and fuse the syllables into a single breath group or phrase on the expiratory phase of respiration.

Abdominal muscle action presents a controlled type of movement, providing a support for the chest muscle action. "Normal speech consists of a series of rapid, highly skilled movements of both the breathing muscles and the muscles of articulation." (23, p. 4.)

Teaching speech to laryngectomized individuals must not only provide functional speech and comply with good mental hygiene principles, but must function within the framework of a satisfactory learning theory involving goal attainment and primary and secondary reinforcements.

This study proposes to investigate the breathing and speech coordinations and articulation efficiency of a group of laryngectomized adults as compared with the breathing and speech coordinations of a group of normal speaking adults. Comparative kymograph tracings of the breathing movements for normal and laryngectomized groups appear to offer a profitable approach to this investigation. Other investigators have employed these procedures. Hudgins (23) as well as Rawlings (46) utilized kymographic recordings in studying the speech breathing coordinations of the deaf. Cypreansen (9) also employed kymographic recordings in studying the breathing and speech coordinations of children with cerebral palsy.

Stetson (55) in 1937, reported a study in which he employed kymographic procedures to measure the breathing and speech coordinations, changes of air pressure in the mouth, and the concomitant pulses of the abdominal and thoracic muscles on several laryngectomized speakers who were employing esophageal speech for communication purposes. After analysis of the results of this experiment he advanced the hypothesis that the chest action for each syllable and the breathing movements for phrasing employed by esophageal speakers were those of normal speech.

This present investigation is designed:

1. to examine Stetson's hypothesis on larger comparative groups of laryngectomized and normal speaking subjects;
2. to study the speech intelligibility of the laryngectomized speakers in relation to their speech coordinations;
3. to determine whether the quantitative intelligibility indexes employed in this study will differentiate between the better and poorer laryngectomized speakers;
4. to examine the hypothesis that laryngectomized speakers who are judged to be most intelligible continue to employ breathing and speech coordinations, articulation and rhythm more like the normal than do those who are judged to be less intelligible;
5. to determine and classify the articulatory errors produced by the laryngectomized speakers;
6. to investigate the relationship of these articulatory errors to speech intelligibility;
7. to determine the effects of rhythm on speech intelligibility;

This study further purports:

1. to obtain an understanding of the speech relearning processes of laryngectomized individuals;
2. to gain an understanding of some of the variables involved in the intelligibility of speech of these individuals.

With more adequate information a positive therapeutic program may possibly be structured which will provide the basis for an effective rehabilitation program for individuals who have undergone laryngectomy.

This study will present in the order listed a consideration of the following aspects of the problem:

1. A review of the literature.
2. Analysis of the kymograph recordings of a group of fifteen laryngectomized and fifteen normal adult speakers.
3. Speech intelligibility information.
4. Analysis of the speech differences found between the breathing and speech coordinations of laryngectomized and normal speakers.

5. Classification of the articulatory errors of the laryngectomized speakers and their relationship to speech intelligibility.
6. Consideration of rhythm as a factor contributing to intelligibility.
7. An interpretation and discussion of the results.
8. Summary and conclusions.
9. Possible implications for therapy and research.

CHAPTER TWO

SURVEY OF THE LITERATURE

A SURVEY OF THE LITERATURE REVEALS THAT THE QUES-
tions concerning: (1) the role of respiration, (2) location of the air
reservoir, (3) site of the pseudo-glottis, in the production of speech after
laryngectomy require further study.

Clarification of these problems would appear to be vital in the structuring of a speech relearning program for the laryngectomized individual.

Kallen observes:

> The importance of respiration in the development of normal voice
> becomes negative under the new conditions caused by the removal of the
> larynx. It is not only useless, but directly hinders the vicarious mechanism
> and causes rapid fatigue. It is the first obstacle for the patient to over-
> come. (32), p. 496.

Stern (54) reported his X-ray breathing observations of ninety-eight
laryngectomized persons whom he had taught to speak. He indicated
that there should be a definite disassociation between the natural act of
respiration and the acquired act of swallowing or aspiration of air. He
believed that if these were performed cojointly, there would be a mask-
ing of the speech by the air escaping from the tracheostomy opening, and
severe coughing would result. Morrison (41) concurred with Stern's
point of view and advocated the learning of this disassociation process
at the outset of therapy.

Burger and Kaiser reported the following in relation to one of the
laryngectomized individuals whom they felt had excellent speech after
laryngectomy.

> It is the positive expiratory pressure in the thorax that expells not
> only air from the lungs through the windpipe, but also the air from the
> esophagus through the pseudo-glottis and the mouth. In reality the speech-
> mechanism of Mr. H. is quite similar to that of the normal man: taking
> in air through expansion of the thorax, giving off air through constriction
> of the thorax. (8), pp. 103-104.

Kallen examined one of Froechel's laryngectomized individuals who
utilized normal respiratory movements to facilitate the phonation
process.

Examination showed him to have a real esophageal voice. At first this pseudo-voice came only after the deglutition of air. After a few weeks the patient could produce it by aspiration into the esophagus, at the same time articulating it into meaningful sounds. Aspiration was accomplished by a jerk like inspiratory movement of the lower part of the thorax and sudden protrusion of the anterior abdominal wall. Graphic registration of these movements showed that the aspiratory and the expiratory sounds corresponded to the movements of normal phonic respiration. On roentgenologic examination the 'act of speech' was shown to possess two phases, both accompanied by sound. In the first, the diaphragm descended with inspiration, the walls of the esophagus diverging as its lumen underwent dilation on filling with air. This was the phase of inspiration-aspiration. The second phase consisted in accent of the diaphragm and expiration. This was accompanied by gradual approximation of the esophageal walls and contraction of the lumen simultaneously with the depletion of its gaseous content. It was the phase of expiration-expulsion. (32), p. 487.

Seeman's eustachian tube examination and X-ray observations permitted him to conclude:

The speaking mechanism of routine esophagus speakers does not essentially differ from that of normal speech, the patients learn to fill the esophagus during a normal inspiration movement with air and to phonate during expiration, in that way they expel the air of the esophagus by contraction of the esophagus walls. (51), p. 294.

Schilling and Binder (49) considered three laryngectomized persons with whom they examined breathing movements by inspection, tape measure and Gutzman's belt pneumograph in the abdominal and thoracic region.

Results for the first two persons indicated that during silent breathing the breath coordinations are abdominal. In inspiration the abdominal expiration takes place one second later than the thorax section. During speech the expiration phases in speaking are often characterized by long expiratory cessations. The breath cessations are not equal in all sections of the breathing apparatus, but represent a strong incongruence between the abdominal and thorax movements. They explain the existence of great irregularity in expansion, rapidity of progress, and the relationships of inspiration and expiration to one another. This behavior did not appear in normal speech breathing curves.

Schilling and Binder (49) also investigated the irregularities and peculiarities of lung breathing during the speech process and their relationship to the pseudo-voice. They felt that such relationship could operate in two ways:

1. Respiration would continue normally and assist the pharynx "pumping" movement.
2. Respiration would be discontinued and therefore serve to weaken the disturbing cannula noise (air issuing from the tracheal stoma opening).

They attacked this problem by recording the air pressures outside the mouth by means of a facial mask, simultaneously with the movements of the abdomen and thorax.

Results revealed instances of both conditions operating. They found that phases of pharyngeal breathing proceed regularly and independently of the lung breathing. They indicated that the pharynx voice changes in no way when the laryngectomized person holds the cannula closed and is asked to arbitrarily discontinue lung breathing.

They concluded that the peculiarities of the thorax and abdominal breathing movements during speaking do not exist for the purpose of assisting the pharynx pumping work, but rather that the frequent expiratory cessations serve to eliminate or to lessen the cannula noise. This function they felt operated below the level of consciousness.

In the same report they cite the results of an examination of another patient which tended to bear out their alternate hypothesis, namely, that in some cases normal respiration continues and actually assists in the production of voice. They claim, nevertheless, that in spite of the assistance role that normal respiration contributes to the production of the voice, there exists marked asynchronism between the abdominal and thoracic breathing movements.

In 1934, Kallen summarized the available information concerning the respiration-phonation controversy up to that time:

1. Types of phonic respiration in laryngectomized persons can be definitely classified.
2. Two main types of phonic respiration seem to predominate. In one the process of breathing is normal. In the other, renewed respiration occurs with each word, often with each syllable; in this type the interference with the new speech mechanism by ordinary vital respiration seems to persist.
3. A number of forms, both mixed and transitional, fall between the two main ones.
4. In a great number of cases the pneumograph provides a clue to the location of the vicarious air chamber and the pseudo-glottis. The lower these two structures lie the more marked the abdominal component of respiration is likely to be. The higher they lie, the more the thoracic element is likely to play a part in the new way of speaking. This follows if one or the other component of respiration serves as an aid in 'expression' of air necessary to activate the pseudo-glottis.

5. The type of phonic respiration in the laryngectomized person may change with time and come to a certain stability only after many years. The change may be connected with the migration of the air chamber and with such factors as concern facilitation of the neuronic pattern. (32), pp. 488-489.

In direct antithesis to disassociation, Stetson commented in 1937:

At first sight the efforts to make the ordinary expiratory movements for speech would seem to be just the wrong thing for oesophageal speech.

But intelligible speech cannot be made with an air supply exerting continuous pressure on the normal larynx or a substitute larynx, although that is a common assumption. The air pressure must fall to zero between the small groups of syllables, and often between syllables, and a separate pressure pulse must be made for each syllable production in the normal respiratory mechanism. Records of excellent oesophageal speech show that the subject breathes just as in normal speech. (57), p. 101.

In the same year Brighton and Boone perpetuated the respiration-phonation controversy and presented roentgenographic studies of laryngectomized subjects to substantiate their position:

During the period of aspiration of air and while talking, breathing is modified or suspended. The necessity for respiration during these periods is one of the most difficult for patients to learn being entirely opposed to the normal cycle of breathing and respiration. (78), p. 582.

Today the controversy over association or disassociation of respiration and phonation continues to provoke speculation. The literature reveals that each investigator has presented evidence to support his hypothesis, consequently the structuring of programs of therapy for these laryngectomized individuals varies within the framework of the different hypothetical bases.

Moreover, further examination of the pertinent literature dealing with the development of speech after laryngectomy reveals a second major controversy, namely, the possible location of the vicarious air chamber. Morrison postulates the requirements of such a chamber for proper functioning:

(a) It must be large enough to contain more than a few cubic centimeters of air. (b) It must be capable of being filled with air at a reasonably quick rate, voluntarily. (c) The contained air must be expelled again under the control of the will. (d) The current of air so expelled must be such that it will be set into vibration as it passes the pseudo-glottis; this is a very important requirement, from which it seems obvious that the air chamber must lie below, i.e., caudal, to the pseudo-glottis.

The possible sites for this air chamber are: . . . the mouth, the pharynx, particularly the hypopharynx, the esophagus as a whole, more especially its upper thoracic and cervical portions, and the cardiac end of the stomach. (41), p. 418.

Stern (53) the strongest advocate of the stomach-air reservoir hypothesis insisted that this phenomenon occurred in the greatest percentage of those laryngectomized individuals he trained to speak. His roentgenographic investigations of the enlargement of the stomach or gastric bubble permitted him to postulate the stomach as the vicarious air chamber. He indicated, however, that the stomach does not take the place of the substituting air reservoir in all cases, but rather frequently the esophagus and the hypopharynx assumes this function. In these individuals he found no appreciable enlargement of the stomach bubble.

He also discussed the "migration of the air reservoir." He observed that during the course of therapy the air reservoir rises constantly higher, with the result that the path of the air, swallowed for the purpose of producing voice, became shortened and eventually the reservoir was to be located in the esophagus or hypopharynx.

In contrast to Stern's work, Seeman (51) concluded that the esophagus because of its psysiological and anatomical construction is predestined to be the substituting air reservoir in the development of speech after laryngectomy. He conducted his experiments on laryngectomized individuals and substantiated previous results which revealed that the esophagus expands during inspiration and contracts during expiration.

Stetson's (55) experiment revealed that the vicarious air chamber was located in the upper part of the esophagus, and that the small reservoir of two to five cc. of air did not enter the stomach. He further noted "that the intake of air is made frequently and rapidly with the mouth and velum closed; it often fuses with the movement of the consonant."

Kallen considered the manner of teaching the laryngectomized to have a direct effect on the location of the air reservoir:

> I believe that the whole matter rests more on the manner of applying the vocal gymnastics than on other factors. Some clinics advocate the swallowing of air, which necessarily is taken down into the stomach. Other clinics advocate the aspiration of air into the esophagus. I have found the latter course much more effective and more practical for the patient. However, the situation is by no means unambiguous. Many of the facts involved are not as yet known and when one method should be preferred to another is still problematic. (32), p. 473.

Morrison introduces a third major controversy by denoting requirements for the proper functioning of the pseudo-glottis.

> (a) It must consist of some portions of the organ concerned that can be set into vibration by the air current passing out of the chamber below; hence it must lie above, i.e., cephaled, to the air chamber. (b) It must be a place that is, or that can be, constricted until the frequency of the vibrations of the passing air current is such that it will yield an audible sound.

(c) It must be under the control of the will in some degree. (d) If the tension of the part or parts that vibrate can be changed at will, the pitch of the resultant sounds will be capable of modulating; . . . (41), p. 418.

Stern experienced difficulty in determining exactly where the site of the pseudo-glottis developed because of the inaccessibility of the structures involved. Nevertheless, he lists the possible areas where its formation might occur:

1. between base of tongue and posterior wall of the pharynx;
2. between the back of the tongue and the tightly stretched velum;
3. between the strongly contracted posterior palatine arches of the two sides;
4. between contracted portions of the inferior constrictor muscle of the pharynx;
5. between the epiglottis and two folds formed laterally from the musculature of the pharynx;
6. at the hiatus of the esophagus, the esophageal mouth of Killian, between folds formed by the cricopharyngeus muscle.
7. In some cases there seems to be no real pseudo-glottis, the patient merely employing the sound produced by the eructation of swallowed air for phonation. (41), p. 418.

Stetson presents a differential construct:

In any form of oesophageal speech the opening of the oesophagus constitutes the substitute glottis. Stern's series of possible locations of the substitute glottis is a physiological phantasy; he loses sight of the necessary use of the tongue and velum in consonant articulation when he places a substitute larynx between the tongue and velum or the tongue and the posterior wall of the pharynx; and a constriction of the muscles of the pharynx to produce a glottis must interfere with the formation of both vowels and consonants. (57), p. 99.

Negus further considered the anatomical and physiological mechanism of the pseudo-glottis and postulated the possibility of the cricopharyngeal sphincter as the possible location of the pseudo-glottis:

When the pharynx is repaired, at the conclusion of the laryngectomy, the constrictor muscle is reunited so that it may regain its ability to contract and to propel food. It is to be presumed that the physiological distinctions between the oblique and circular fibres remain, to a certain extent, and that a sphincter is thus reformed at the mouth of the esophagus. Apparently it has less control over the entrance of air than in the normal individual and so air-swallowing becomes easy. . . . It appears probable that the constriction formed by the sphincter may even act as a reed and may thus be the origination of sound, for use in speech. (42), pp. 855-856.

Lindsey, Morgan and Wepman employed roentgenologic techniques on laryngectomized persons and reported that proficiency of esophageal voice seems to be dependent on the ability of the individual to control the cricopharyngeus muscle. They describe the phonation process:

The pharynx dilates with air, the sphincter opens with flash-like sudden-
ness, allowing air to pass into the upper end of the esophagus, accompanied
in the less proficient by a slight sound. The air can then be immediately
utilized for production of voice.

As air passes into the esophagus there is also inspiration of a small amount
of air into the trachea. During speech the abdominal muscles contract, the
diaphragm rises and air is exhaled from the trachea as well as through the
pharynx. In the accomplished subject the interchange of air both in the
trachea and pharynx during speech is quite limited. During phonation, the
column of air in the pharynx is narrowed anteroposteriorly but the base
of the tongue remains well separated from the posterior pharyngeal wall
and does not show evidence of vibratory motion. (37), pp. 63-64.

Stetson (57), Negus (42), Lindsey, Morgan, and Wepman (37) agree
that the probable site of the pseudo-glottis lies at the upper portion of
the esophagus.

Anderson (1) in 1950 investigated a number of phenomena of esophageal speech and their relationship to intelligibility. His subjects
comprised twelve laryngectomized individuals who had already learned
esophageal speech.

The investigation dealt with the relationship of intelligibility and:
(1) rate of speaking intelligibility lists, (2) volume of air used in
speech, (3) intensity, (4) number of sounds produced acceptably. Anderson manifested further interest in the relationships of: (1) esophageal vital capacity and the volume of air used in speech, (2) standard
reading time and esophageal reading time, (3) synchronization of intake of air into the mouth with movements of the thorax and abdomen.
Anderson also investigated the esophageal speaker's ability to produce
different sounds. His instrumentation included a small wet spirometer,
two one-way bottle valves, two electric pneumopolygraphs, two girdle-
type pneumographs and a magnecorder. He employed a modified civil-
ian type gas mask which was securely fastened over the subject's face
while he was speaking. The gas mask was modified so that a crystal
microphone was placed in the mouthpiece which was then plugged into
the magnecorder. And the tube which originally led to the canister was
replaced with a funnel which was attached to the mask proper with
rubber cement so that the connection was airtight. The funnel led to
the one-way bottle valves to measure the intake and outflow of air. Poly-
graph tracings provided measurements of this intake and outflow of air.
The pneumographs were placed around the thorax and the abdomen to
record pressure variations at those points.

For speech materials Anderson used the Harvard Phonetically Balanced words (22), Haagen's multiple choice test (21), and Walker's equated five-syllable phrases (63) (equated as to time and intensity). As the subject read the multiple choice list, simultaneous recordings were made of the speech, volume of air, and movements of the abdomen and thorax. The PB words and the five-syllable phrases were recorded on the magnetic tape recorder. He used twelve listeners as judges for the multiple choice intelligibility phrases, and the esophageal speakers were ranked on the basis of the percentage of words understood. For the PB words three judges phonetically transcribed the speaker's responses. These were then analyzed for the purpose of evaluating difficulty levels for the sounds produced. He took X-rays of the esophagus and stomach areas for each speaker, one following a maximal inspiration of air and the other following maximal expiration while the subject phonated a sustained "ah" sound.

On the basis of his analysis, Anderson concluded:

1. Esophageal speakers differ among themselves in intelligibility.
2. Those elements of esophageal speech which appear to be directly related to high intelligibility are (1) intensity, (2) number of sounds produced correctly, and (3) duration of phonation. Those elements which do not appear to be directly related to high intelligibility are: (1) rate of speaking, (2) volume of air used, and (3) esophageal vital capacity.
3. The volume of air used by esophageal speakers in speaking is small and is stored in the esophagus. The range among the speakers extended from an amount too small to measure to 18.055 cc. per word with a mean of 9.485 cc. No specific amount was found which could be recommended as optimum.
4. Although great variation was noted from speaker to speaker three relationships are apparent with reference to intake of air into the mouth and movement of the abdomen and thorax. These are: (1) fixation of the respiratory movements of the abdomen and thorax takes place during the intake of air into the esophagus. (2) intake of air into the mouth is neither significantly synchronous or asynchronous with inspiratory movements of the abdomen and thorax. (3) Generally speaking the abdomen and thorax exhibit synchrony of gross patterns if the record is inspected as a whole, but this synchrony does not exist if the tracings are compared for small detail.
5. Some sounds are more difficult than others for the esophageal speaker to produce intelligibly. (1), pp. 92-93.

Anderson's results appear to substantiate the hypothesis as stated by Kallen (32) in his review of the research, i.e., that the lower the pseudo-glottis is, the more marked the abdominal component of respiration is likely to be. The higher the pseudo-glottis is, the greater is the thoracic element.

As late as 1952, Bateman, Dornhorst, and Leathart (5) reported observations concerning the location of the vicarious air chamber and the site of the pseudo-glottis on three patients who had undergone complete laryngectomies and who had well-developed oesophageal speech. The investigators employed a polythene tube of about 1 mm. external and 0.5 mm. internal diameter with two or three lateral holes near one end. The end was passed through the nose into the esophagus. The free end was attached to a capacitance manometer, and the system was filled with water. In recording trunk expansion a length of "elephant" tubing was lightly strapped around the chest and another around the abdomen. The two lengths were joined by a "Y" connection to a second manometer, which recorded the decrease in pressure produced by stretching the tubing. The fluoroscopic technique was employed for examination of the subjects. Barium paste was utilized to outline the esophageal walls. All three subjects gave substantially similar results.

They outlined the following processes of phonation:

The cricopharyngeal sphincter is kept closed until the patient is about to speak. He then releases it, allowing the oesophagus to fill, which it readily does because of the negative intra-thoracic pressure to which it is exposed. The rate of filling being further enhanced by a simultaneous respiratory movement. The patient then closes the sphincter and raises the intra-thoracic pressure by a sharp expiratory effort. The rise in oesophageal pressure forces some air through the sphincter, causing a sound which is then modulated by tongue movement in the usual way. The effective lower limit of the air reservoir is the diaphragm and not the cardia. Although some air enters the stomach, this is a side effect and there is no evidence that stomach air is belched out to form the speech sound. (5), p. 1177.

The most extensive research at the present time specifically related to the articulatory errors and their relationship to the intelligibility of laryngectomized speakers has been done by Anderson (1) and Hyman (29).

Anderson investigated the effect of articulatory errors on the speech intelligibility of laryngectomized individuals. His sample included twelve laryngectomized individuals all of whom employed speech without mechanical means. The criterion used for evaluating articulatory efficiency was the Harvard Phonetically Balanced Lists (22). Three judges transcribed phonetically the person's responses. These transcriptions were analyzed to determine the errors in the sound categories. The sounds were categorized first as consonants and vowels. The consonants were further classified as voiced and voiceless, nasals, stop-plosives, semivowels, fricatives and glides. Anderson concluded:

1. Esophageal speakers produce some sounds more intelligibly than others. Sounds listed from most to least intelligible have the following order: a) vowels, b) laterals, c) glides, d) nasals, e) voiced consonants, f) initial consonants, g) stop-plosives, h) final consonants, i) voiceless consonants and j) fricatives.
2. The number of sounds produced intelligibly were significantly related to high intelligibility scores. (1), p. 91.

Hyman (29) also investigated the effect of articulatory errors on intelligibility for three groups. He selected: (1) good laryngectomized speakers who employed the artificial larynx, (2) good laryngectomized speakers who used no mechanical means, (3) normal speakers.

The criterion employed by Hyman to determine speech intelligibility was lists of words from Haagen's multiple-choice intelligibility test (21). The articulatory errors were derived from performance on a monosyllabic test (29). Seven persons transcribed phonetically the speakers' responses. The responses of the auditors were analyzed to obtain the errors that were produced for each sound category. The sounds of the monosyllabic test were categorized into consonants and vowels. The consonants were further subdivided into voiced and voiceless, initial and final and then plosive, fricative, affricative, nasals and glides. Hyman concluded:

1. The vowel sounds for all three groups of speakers were identified more times than consonants.
2. There was a significant difference in preference among college students of voices, loudness levels, and duration of reading of artificial larynx and esophageal speakers. This difference was in favor of the artificial-larynx speakers. (29), p. 115.

The sounds listed from most to least intelligible for the esophageal speakers have the following order: (1) vowels, (2) affricatives, (3) glides, (4) nasals, (5) plosives, (6) voiced consonants, (7) initial consonants, (8) final consonants, (9) voiceless consonants, (10) fricatives, (29).

Anderson (1) and Hyman (29) considered sound categories in recording errors rather than types of errors produced.

The controversies emanating from this research are not due to a paucity of studies, but rather to the failure of a large number of investigators attacking the problem from various points of view.

A few scholars, primarily physicians, have conducted prodigious research, but in most cases their investigations have been influenced mainly by their specific interests. Research was principally related to the laryngectomized individuals whom they had taught to speak, and was designed and devoted to the development of a theoretical structure for testing the efficacy of their therapy. Most of these studies failed to provide adequate controls against the experimental variables.

The present investigation purports to study:

1. the breathing and speech coordinations of laryngectomized speakers who were not instructed in any one therapeutic framework;

2. a sample of normal speakers as controls. The comparisons resulting from the study should contribute to the clarification of the prevalent controversial issues.

3. a variety of speech materials to arrive at intelligibility indexes which will be specifically related to the breathing and speech coordinations;

4. the effect of articulatory errors and rhythm on speech intelligibility;

5. in addition to the comparisons between the laryngectomized and normal subjects, comparisons within the laryngectomized group should also contribute important insights to the speech re-learning process.

CHAPTER THREE

EXPERIMENTAL DESIGN AND PROCEDURES

THE FOLLOWING EXPERIMENTAL DESIGN, INSTRUMEN-
tation, materials, subjects and procedures were utilized in investigating
the breathing and speech coordinations of laryngectomized and normal
subjects, and the relationships between the breathing and speech coordinations and articulatory errors to the speech intelligibility of
laryngectomized subjects.

INSTRUMENTATION

THE KYMOGRAPH

A variable-speed, motor-driven, custom-built kymograph, carrying
Western Union Teledeltos paper eight inches wide, was employed
throughout the experiment. The paper was fed through the kymograph
by a friction-driven mechanism operating two gears. The breathing and
speech movements and the air pressure developed by these movements
were transmitted to the paper by means of pneumodeiks. The pneumodeik is sensitive to pressure changes and makes possible comparisons
of air pressure tracings over variable time periods.

The efficacy of the pneumodeik as a reliable measuring device in
pneumatic recording has been reported previously by Hudgins and
Stetson (28). Similar pneumodeiks were employed in this investigation.

The following factors were checked carefully before, during and after
each session of kymograph recordings in the present study: (1) timing
apparatus, (2) alignment of recording styli, (3) the excursion arcs of
the recording styli in response to known applied pressures.

The subjects stood erect in a wooden stanchion during the kymograph tracings. Figure 1 is a photograph of the entire apparatus employed for these tracings. [The apparatus in use was similar to that
used by Hudgins as employed in the investigations of the speech coordinations of the deaf (23)]. The back upright of the frame had two
adjustable bearing points (wooden blocks) which were adjusted so
that the subject was supported at the thoracic and lumbar spine points.

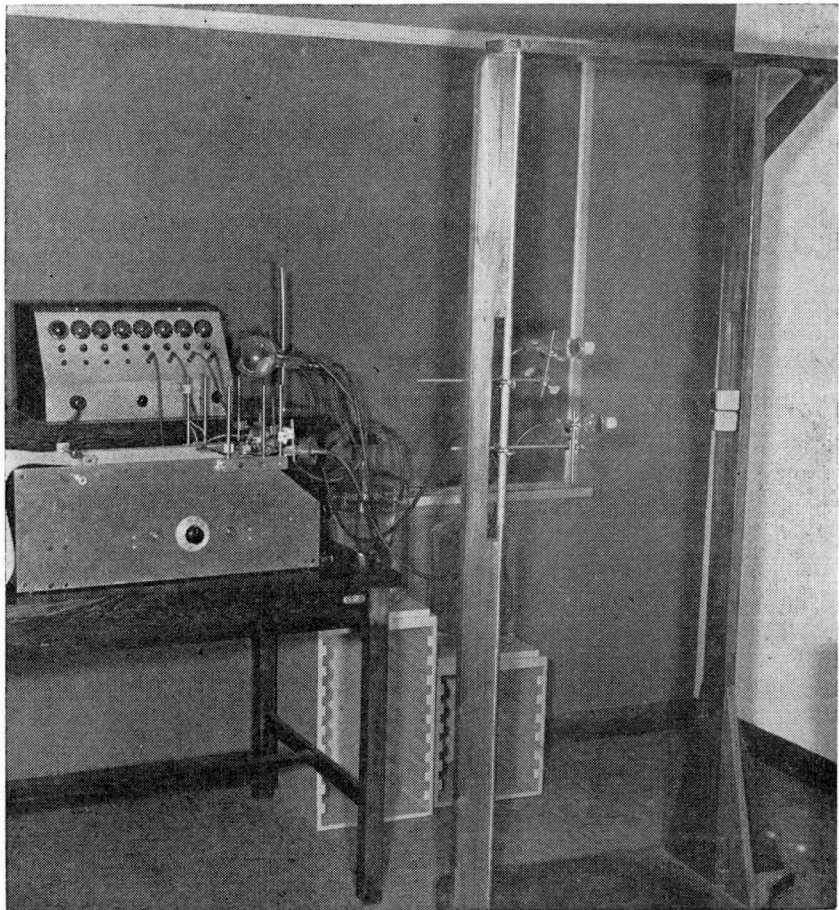

Fig. 1. Illustration of the apparatus employed in measuring breathing and speech coordinations showing the high voltage rectifier, the variable speed kymograph, the negative pressure apparatus, and the wooden stanchion.

This arrangement prevented any backward movement during the recording of the kymograph tracings. A half-inch pipe fitted to the edge of a four-inch board, formed the upright in front of the subject and held the recording tambours independently of the subject. This arrangement permitted the tambours to be moved into any desired position so that any particular area of the subject's body could be explored and recorded.

The upright frame wherein the subject stood was six feet high and twenty-six inches wide. The apparatus was designed to avoid hampering the subject unduly, but at the same time to fixate the trunk at the necessary points.

Thistle tube recording tambours two inches in diameter were applied to the body wall. The open end of each tube was covered with tightly stretched thin rubber. Cork bosses one inch in depth and one and one-fourth inches in diameter were glued to the center of the rubber diaphragms. The tambours were adjusted to the body area to be explored after the subject had been placed in position. The bosses were then pressed against the body wall until the rubber diaphragms were forced into the cup of the thistle tube about half the length of the bosses. As the body wall moved in and out, the bosses were moved in and out, displacing the column of air within the closed recording system. The pressure changes were then transmitted through rubber hoses to two pneumodeiks.

A negative pressure apparatus [similar to that used by Stetson (56) and Hudgins (23)] consisting of a plastic funnel, fitting the contour of the body wall, and having a hose leading to a third pneumodeik, was placed over the epigastric area for the recording of the syllable pulse. The positive stroke of the stylus indicated the beginning of the syllable pulses. A timing stylus, connected to the synchronous motor, recorded time in one-tenth second intervals. The stainless steel writing styli, wrapped with copper wire, were supplied with direct current from a variable high voltage rectifier. Figure 2 illustrates the negative pressure apparatus with the plastic applicator for measurement of the syllable pulse.

In addition, air pressure changes in the mouth, outside the mouth, and simultaneous tracings of the air pressure inside and outside of the mouth were recorded. Changes of the air pressure in the mouth (A.I.) behind the consonant occlusion were obtained by a metal tube with a lumen one millimeter in diameter. In order to allow the articulatory organs freedom of movement, the metal tube was shaped and curved to fit the corner of the mouth and to pass back to the rear of the mouth paralleling the teeth. A sharp bend near the end of the tube permitted it to enter the oral cavity proper around the last molar and to rest in a position in the region of the oral pharynx.

The air pressure just outside the mouth (A.O.) was recorded by means of a rubber "embouchure" shaped to fit the contour of the mouth. A small hole ventilated the "embouchure." In order to obtain the combined pressure, the metal tube was inserted in the rubber "em-

bouchure." Rubber tubes connected to the metal tube and the "embouchure" led individually to the respective pneumodeiks.

The sub-glottal variations of the air pressure were obtained by enclosing the tracheal stoma in a rubber concave embouchure. A hole in
the embouchure permitted rubber tubing to be inserted which led to
the respective recording pneumodeiks. The arrangement was such that
the laryngectomized individual was in complete control of the mask for
breathing purposes.

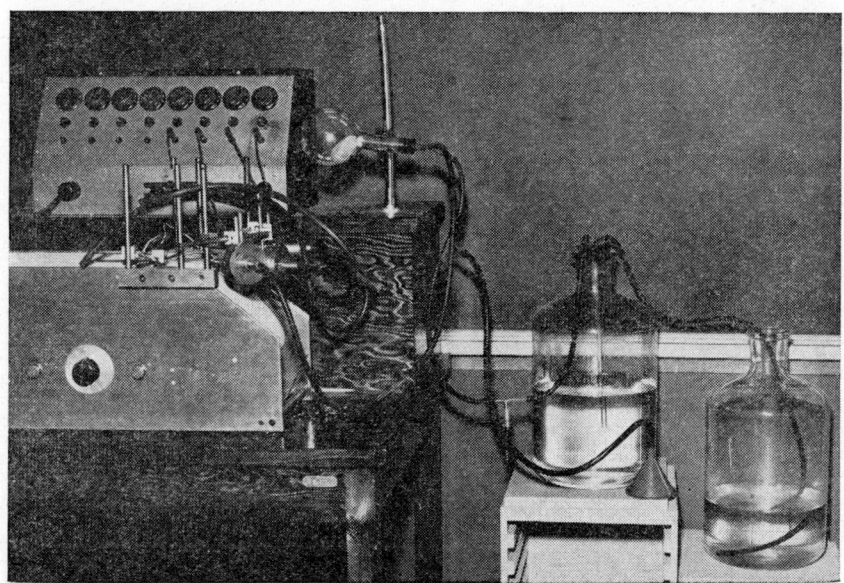

FIG. 2. Illustration of the negative pressure apparatus including the plastic
applicator, the variable speed kymograph, and the high voltage rectifier are
also shown for measurement of the syllable pulse.

THE MAGNECORDER

The Magnecorder, Model PT 6-J and A H, was employed for tape
recording the speech samples. The subjects, by preference, stood in
front of and spoke into a Shure cardiod floor-stand microphone placed
at a distance of approximately nine inches from the speaker's mouth.
The cardiod microphone is relatively insensitive to small changes in
azimuth and speaking distance.

A trained technician monitored the recording level of the Magnecorder by means of a standard volume indicator. A sound-treated room
sixteen by eighteen feet, suspended by springs from the frame of the

building and treated with glass wool and perforated transite, was utilized in making the recordings. The floor was covered with rubber matting and carpeting. The ambient sound level of the room was lower than could be measured with a General Radio Sound-level Meter set at position A.

A portion of the taped material was transferred to twelve-inch acetate discs to facilitate play-back and analysis. The output of the Magnecorder was fed directly to a Rek-o-Kut cutting head through conventional matching transformer and equalizing network. The disc recordings were made at seventy-eight revolutions per minute on a Rek-o-Kut turntable.

MEASURING DEVICE FOR THE KYMOGRAPH TRACINGS

A special device was constructed for measuring the kymograph tracings. Figure 3 shows a movable parallel straight edge placed at the bottom of a drawing board twenty by twenty-six inches in size, with a lower bar securely fastened on an even edge with the bottom of the board. This left the upper bar capable of sliding up and down on the hinges, forming a parallel base line anywhere between three and six inches above the base of the board. When the kymograph tracings were slipped beneath the straight edge, it was possible to make an accurate base line for any cycle to be measured.

A narrow edge of wood was cemented parallel and even with the bottom edge of the seventy millimeter, transparent plastic triangle. This

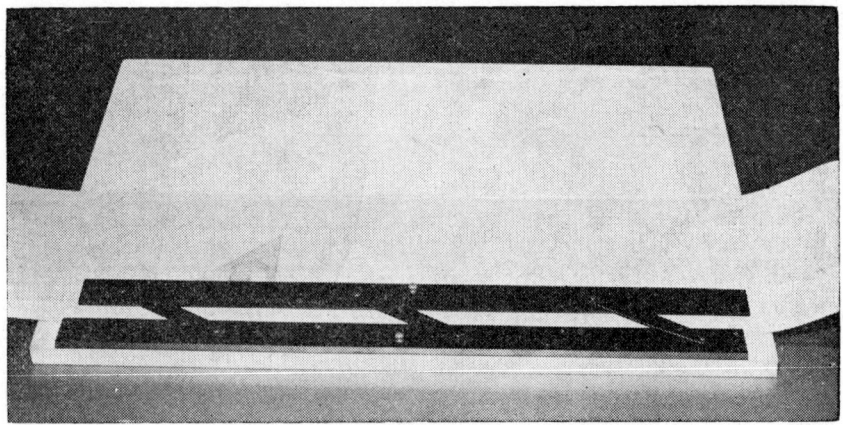

FIG. 3. Illustration of the measuring device used on the kymograph tracings showing the adjustable parallel straight edge and the millimeter triangle used in the measurement of amplitude.

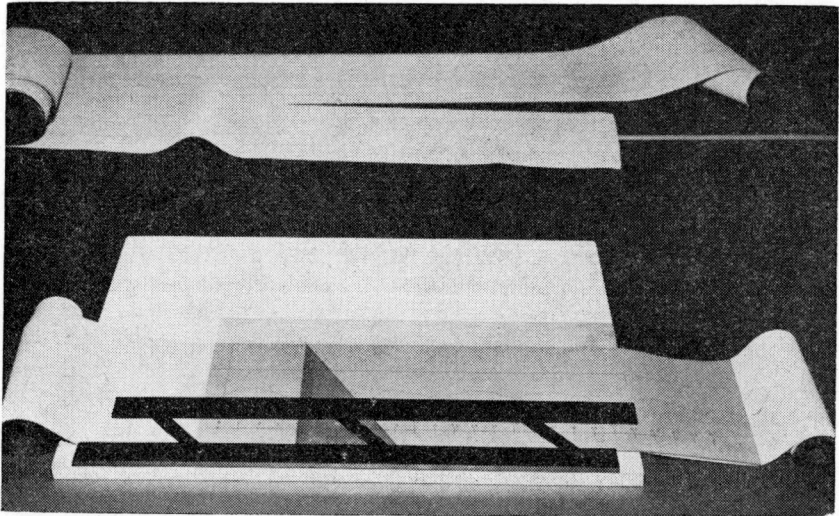

Fig. 4. Illustration of the measuring device used on the kymograph tracings showing the plastic sheet marked in seconds and the large right-angle triangle for measurement of time.

triangle, when placed against the movable straight edge, could be moved to form a base line at the lowest point at the beginning of the cycle to be measured. Figure 3 also illustrates how this provided accurate measuring of the amplitude of the cycles to the nearest half millimeter.

A heavy transparent plastic sheet, eleven by twenty-six inches, was marked off in time intervals of one second to match the ten one-tenth seconds speed of the kymograph tracings. The plastic sheet was also marked with a perpendicular line at the zero point. This line was moved to the beginning of each unit to be measured in time. An eight-inch transparent millimeter triangle formed a right-angle line at the end of the time unit, providing the making of accurate time measurements at the same time the amplitude measurements were being made. Figure 4 illustrates the time measurement apparatus.

The reliability of the instrument as a measuring device for amplitude was determined by having five graduate students in speech pathology and audiology each make fifty measurements on the same kymograph tracings of normal and laryngectomized speakers in silence and speech. The experimenter's consistency in measuring amplitude with this instrument was determined by making a series of five independent readings of these same fifty tracings.

Table 56 in the appendix reveals the substantial degree of agreement for the amplitude measurements in millimeters for the five readers and for the series of readings by the experimenter. Reliability coefficients were computed for readers A and B (.9989) and C and D (.9992) ; and between experimenter measurements 2 and 5 (.9992).

SUBJECTS

The normal-speaking subjects included in this study were fifteen male residents of Syracuse, New York, between the ages of thirty-seven and seventy years, with a mean age of 60.1 years and a median age of 59. These normal subjects who volunteered to participate in the study represented several occupational areas.

The fifteen laryngectomized subjects who participated in the study were males between the ages of thirty-six and seventy-four years, with a mean age of 59.9 years and a median age of 60.5 years. Ten of the laryngectomized speakers living in Syracuse, New York were reached through the cooperative efforts of local laryngologists or through the facilities of the Gordon D. Hoople Hearing and Speech Center of Syracuse University. Three of these ten speakers had received speech training at the University Center. The remaining five laryngectomized speakers resided in other cities in New York State and were recommended as subjects for the study by various laryngologists over the State.[1]

Each of the fifteen laryngectomized speakers employed phonated speech for communication purposes without the use of any type of artificial larynx. All of the members of both the normal and the laryngectomized groups had normal hearing and the normal speakers were free from any observable speech deviations.

The laryngologists who were the first to approach each subject, described the nature and purpose of the investigation and explained that no medical risk would be involved through participation in the study.

After the initial orientation by the laryngologists, the experimenter met with each laryngectomized person who had agreed to cooperate in the experiment, and arrangements were completed for participation in the study.

---

[1]See Tables 52 and 53 in the Appendix for further identifying information in regard to the normal and laryngectomized speakers.

THE MATERIALS OF THE STUDY

FOR THE KYMOGRAPH RECORDINGS

The materials employed for the kymograph recordings of the speech breathing movements of the normal and laryngectomized subjects consisted of a sixty-syllable paragraph and phrases of five, seven, and nine syllables. In addition, six groups of four syllables consisting of releasing and arresting consonants were included. The fifth group in this series possessed neither releasing nor arresting consonants. A seventh group comprising eight syllables broken into four groups of two syllables each; the first containing a releasing consonant, and the second containing neither a releasing nor an arresting consonant.

The speech materials as listed below were typed on white cards four by six inches in size.

1. The sixty-syllable paragraph:
   IN THE AUTUMN OF THE YEAR WHEN THE WEATHER GETS COLD MOST OF THE BIRDS FLY SOUTH. IF THEY DID NOT GO SOUTH THEY WOULD NOT FIND ENOUGH FOOD TO EAT. WHEN THEY DO NOT HAVE ENOUGH FOOD TO EAT THEY WILL BE COLD. FOOD IS QUITE NECESSARY TO KEEP THEM WARM.

2. The five-syllable phrase:
   MOTHER BAKED A CAKE.

3. The seven-syllable phrase:
   HE WENT HOME IN THE SNOWSTORM.

4. The nine-syllable phrase.
   THE MAN PUT THE BOOK ON THE TABLE.

5. The four-syllable phrases:
   a. [bʌ]   [bʌ]   [bʌ]   [bʌ]
   b. [pʌ]   [pʌ]   [pʌ]   [pʌ]
   c. [ʌb]   [ʌb]   [ʌb]   [ʌb]
   d. [ʌp]   [ʌp]   [ʌp]   [ʌp]
   e. [ɑ]   [ɑ]   [ɑ]   [ɑ]
   f. [hɑ]   [hɑ]   [hɑ]   [hɑ]
   g. [hɑ-ɑ]   [hɑ-ɑ]   [hɑ-ɑ]   [hɑ-ɑ]

THE TAPE RECORDINGS

The speech materials[2] for the Magnecorder tape recordings used in measuring the intelligibility of the laryngectomized speakers consisted of:

_____

[2]Samples of the speech materials appear in the Appendix.

1. Fifteen different lists of fifty phonetically balanced monosyllabic words (14).

   These fifteen lists were randomly selected from a group of twenty, and the words for each of the fifteen lists were then randomly selected by means of a table of random numbers.

2. Fifteen different twenty-four-word multiple choice tests (21) equated as to difficulty. The fifteen tests were randomly selected from the available twenty-four equivalent tests. Each test consisted of twenty-four words read in groups of three.

3. Ten unrelated, different sentences for each speaker.

   The sentences contained from four to eleven syllables, with a mean of seven syllables for the one hundred and fifty sentences. The sentences were typewritten on four by six-inch cards. Difficult and unfamiliar words or complicated grammatical construction were avoided. No attempt was made to "load" the sentences with specific sounds. An analysis was made of the phonetic content of the sentences and this was compared to Dewey's list of the relative frequencies of the speech sounds (11).[3] Although there were some differences in the ranking and percentages of the frequencies of sounds, those sounds used the most frequently in the present study follow Dewey's list in close approximation. The fifteen sets of ten sentences were checked for reliability of testing speech intelligibility by means of the split-half method corrected for length. A correlation of .96 was obtained.

THE PROCEDURES OF THE STUDY

THE KYMOGRAPH RECORDINGS

Previous to the actual recording the normal and the laryngectomized subjects were instructed, during the individual interviews with the experimenters, in the procedures of the kymograph recording. A period of practice followed the period of instruction. This orientation allowed the subject to become familiar with the equipment, the speech materials and the specific procedures of the experiment. The time in amount of practice varied for each individual in relation to the time needed to secure adequate adjustment to the recording situation and gain ease and confidence in the speaking situation.

After the subject had indicated that he was ready, he took his place in erect position in the stanchion, and the thoracic and lumbar wooden

---

[3]The comparison of the phonetic content with Dewey's norms appears in the Appendix, Table 57.

block bearing points were adjusted for the experimental recording. The blocks fixated the trunk at these critical points and the tracings of the body wall movements could then be made with the use of the thistle tube tambours and the bosses.

One tambour was placed at the lower sternum area to record the rib cage movements, the other at the mesogastric area to record the movements of the body wall in the abdominal region. The funnel, a part of the negative pressure apparatus, was then placed in position for the recording of the syllable pulse. Figures 5 and 6 show the equipment and the subject in position for the kymograph recording.

Kymograph recordings for the normal and the laryngectomized subjects were secured as follows:

1. Movements in silent breathing, one minute duration:
   Instructions to the subject:
   > During the next minute you will stand as still as possible. Do not speak during this time. Look straight in front of you. You will be signaled when this portion of the recording is completed.

2. Movements in speech breathing:
   Instructions to the subject:
   > The speech material which you are to read is the same as that which you have previously practiced. Signal when you wish to begin. When you have completed the paragraph, we will stop. When you are ready to begin the phrases which come next, you will signal to us again. The same procedures will continue through the reading of the groups of four syllables.

   The speech material, typed on cards, was placed before the subject on the upright of the stanchion at proper eye level. When the subject indicated he was ready to begin, the sixty-syllable paragraph; the five, seven and nine syllable phrases; and the groups of four syllable phrases were spoken, and the respective movements of the body wall were recorded on the kymograph. The kymograph tracings were marked as each subject completed each part of the speech recording.

3. Tracings of air pressure outside of the mouth: The fitted embouchure was applied over the subject's mouth. The speech material for this part of the study consisted of phrases of five, seven, nine and four syllables in length.

4. Tracings of the air pressure inside the mouth: The same material which was employed in the tracings of the air pressure outside of the mouth were used in this part of the study. To secure the air pressure inside the mouth, the specially constructed metal tube was used.

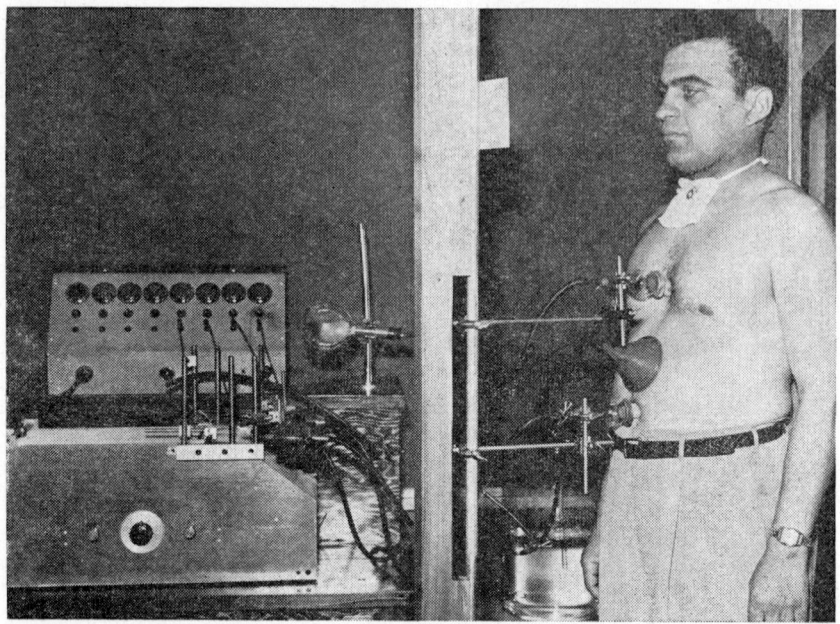

Fig. 5. Illustration of apparatus with laryngectomized subject in position for recording of speech breathing coordinations, showing the two recording tambours applied to the body wall at the lower sternum area and at the mesogastric area, with the negative pressure applicator for the recording of the syllable pulse also in position.

5. Securing the combined air pressure tracings: The metal tube was placed through a small opening in the embouchure and the air pressure inside and outside the mouth were recorded simultaneously, using the same speech material as used in 3 and 4 above.

6. Tracings of the syllable pulse and the sub-glottal air pressures: Simultaneous recordings were made of the tracings of the syllable pulse and sub-glottal air pressures. The negative pressure applicator (funnel) was applied to the epigastric area for the recording of the syllable pulses. The sub-glottal pressure was secured by means of a rubber embouchure shaped to the contour of the neck and placed over the tracheal stoma.

The purpose of this part of the experiment was to discover the relationship of the syllable pulse to the escape of sub-glottal air. A similar procedure was employed by Stetson (57). The subjects understood that they were in complete control of the rubber embouchure held over the tracheal stoma. This could be removed at any time if the subject desired.

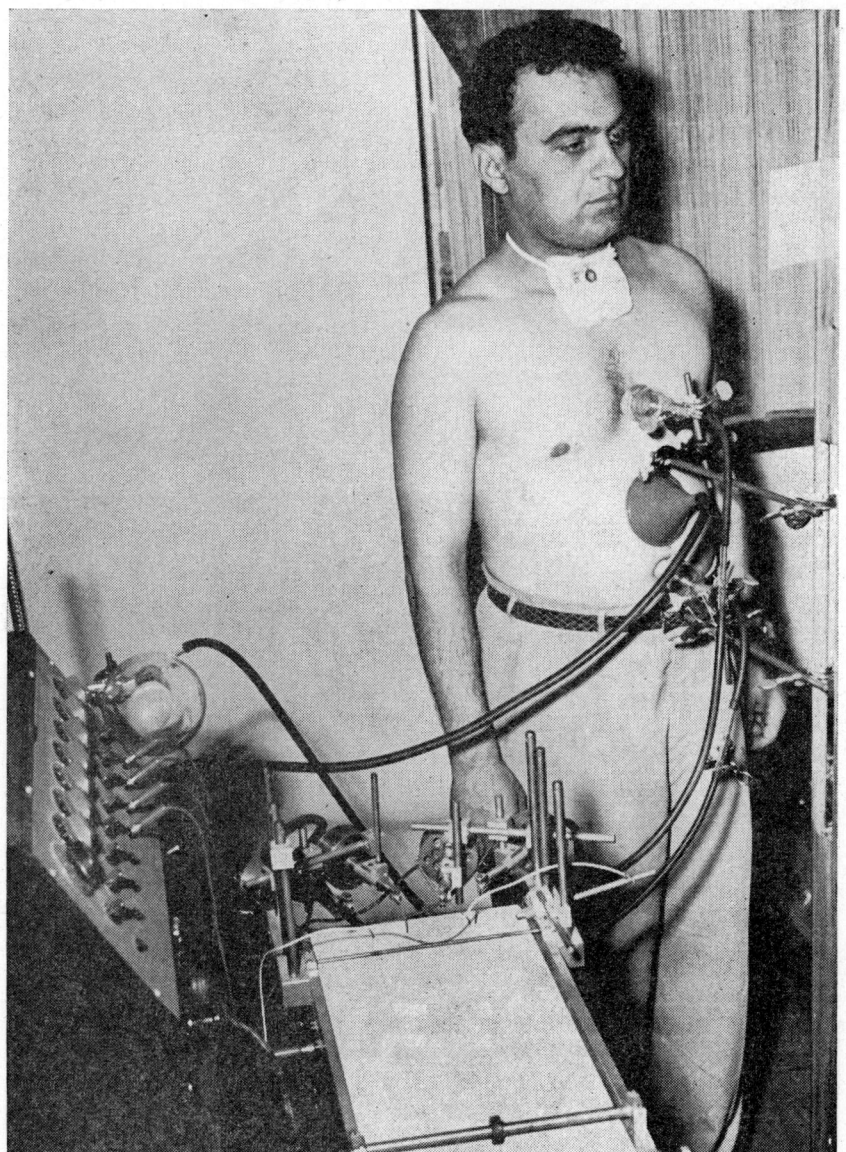

FIG. 6. Illustration of apparatus with laryngectomized subject in position for recording of speech breathing coordinations, showing the two recording tambours applied to the body wall at the lower sternum area and at the mesogastric area, with the negative pressure applicator for the recording of the syllable pulse also in position; also indicating the kymograph, sensitive pneumodeiks, writing styli, and Western Union teledeltos paper.

The speech material for this part of the study was the same as that used in the tracings of the pressure outside and inside of the mouth in 3 and 4 above. With the negative pressure applicator (the funnel) in position and the rubber embouchure held over the tracheal stoma, the pressure of the sub-glottal air was recorded.

The Tape Recordings for the Laryngectomized Subjects

The tape recordings of the speech of the laryngectomized subjects were made in a sound-treated room. Figure 7 illustrates the equipment and the recording position of the subject. The subjects were given an opportunity to become familiar with the speech material and the recording procedures.

The speaker stood in front of and spoke into a Shure cardioid floor microphone placed at a distance of approximately nine inches from the speaker's mouth. The standing position was selected as the preferred position by the subjects.

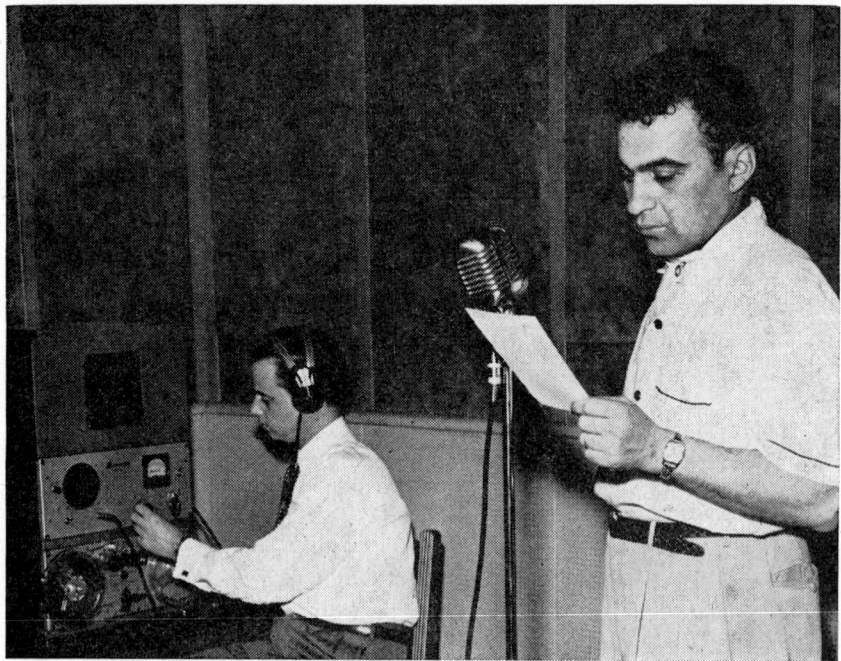

Fig. 7. Illustration of laryngectomized subject in sound-treated room, in position for speech recording, showing Magnecorder, cardioid floor stand microphone, and technician in position for monitoring tape recording.

The following instructions were given to each subject at the time of the final recording:

I shall give you typewritten cards of the different speech materials that we shall use in recording your speech. You have already practiced this material. When you are ready for the first card you will signal so that the operator can begin the recording. The first card contains fifty words. When the operator signals, I will wait a few seconds and then will say, 'number 1.' After a brief pause you will say the first word. When the operator signals again I will say, 'number 2.' You will follow by saying the second word, and continue until you have completed the fifty words. If at any time you wish to stop, you will signal. Feel free to stop as often as you wish. The second card will contain eight three-word groups. We shall stop after each three words. We shall resume recording when you signal. The last card will contain the ten sentences, and we shall follow the same procedure as for the preceding two cards. We shall stop after each sentence and then wait for your signal to begin again. Are there any questions?

The tape recordings were spaced in time and periods of silence for the purpose of facilitating and expediting the auditing procedures.

THE AUDITING PROCEDURES

Two types of auditors were utilized in this study: (1) A group of speech pathology and audiology majors, (2) A group of non-speech pathology and audiology majors.

The auditors had normal hearing. A sound-treated room, twenty-one by sixteen feet in size, removed from street noise, was employed for auditing. Before each auditing period the room was measured for its ambient noise level with a General Radio Sound-level Meter, Type 759-B. An approximate noise level of thirty-eight decibels was found. The auditors preferred to listen at a seventy decibel level.

A high fidelity, custom-built play-back containing a Permoflux speaker was employed to play back the disc recordings which had been transferred from the tape recordings. The measured response of the complete play-back system was electrically flat from 100 to 6,000 cycles. The part of the tape recordings not transferred to discs was played back on the Magnecorder employing an eight-inch Permoflux, high-fidelity speaker adequately baffled. The Permoflux speaker comes very close to reproducing the entire frequency range of the tape. The reported range of this speaker is from 50 to 13,000 cycles.

The net result of monitoring both the original tapes and the dubbing of the discs was to equalize levels within the limitations of the monitor and the conventional volume indicator.

The following instructions were read to the auditors and mimeographed audition scoring sheets were provided for each part of the recorded speech material.[4]

The lists of phonetically balanced words and the multiple choice intelligibility test list were played back one time only. Each sentence in the lists of ten sentences was played back three times. The directions for auditing the phonetically balanced word lists were as follows:

> You will hear a series of fifty words. Each word will be played just once. You will be given time for writing between the presentation of the words. After hearing each word, write down in the properly numbered space the word you think you hear. If you are not certain of the word, make a guess, but do not guess wildly. If you are completely uncertain of the word, you may leave the space blank, and continue to the writing of the next word. . . . Are there any questions?

The following directions were given for auditing Haagen's Multiple Choice Lists according to his instructions:

> Look at the words carefully and be certain to draw a line through . . . the word that you think was read. In some cases there is a difference of only a single letter, so make your selection carefully. Also remember that only one of the four words is correct. If two words within a single group of four are marked, it is an error. If you have marked a word and then decide that that choice is wrong, write the word *no* beside it. The first word that is read is always in the column to the left. The second word is always in the center column, and the third word is always in the column to the right. For each [speaker] begin with the first set of choice words and continue down the page in order. Be careful to make a heavy mark . . . through the word. [Have you any questions?]

The following directions were given for auditing the sentences:

> You will hear ten sentences. Each sentence will be played three times. Write what you think the sentence was the first time you hear it in the space provided. The first hearing of the first sentence is numbered 1-a. Write what you think you hear on the second playing of the first sentence in the space numbered 1-b, and so on. Do not change the writing of any sentence; you may change the writing of the second playing, if the second playing makes a difference in the sentence. If you are not quite sure, guess, but do not make wild guesses. If the sentence is completely lacking in intelligibility, you may leave the space blank. . . . Are there any questions?

The members of the auditing group changed at each auditing session. Eighty-four different individuals served as auditors at different periods. The number of auditors at any one time ranged from seven to fifteen. The minimum auditing group at any time was seven in number and always included at least five speech pathology and audiology majors. The auditors were seated comfortably around a large table.

[4]Copies of the auditing sheets appear in the Appendix.

The auditing period lasted approximately two hours, with a break of ten minutes between each hour. Eighteen evenings were given to auditing. The evening was selected as providing the most optimum time for auditing, since at this time the auditors were available and the building was quiet.

SYSTEM OF GRADING AUDITING SHEETS

The auditors were provided with prepared auditing sheets. The fifty phonetically balanced words were scored according to the percentage of words correctly understood. Each word understood correctly received two percentage points. The Haagen Multiple Choice Lists were also scored on the basis of percentage of words correctly understood, and Haagen's conversion table formula was employed to arrive at the intelligibility score. The sentences were graded as follows:

1. 10 points were given if the sentence was heard correctly on the first listening.
2. 5 points were given if the sentence was heard correctly on the second repeated listening.
3. 2 points were given if the sentence was heard correctly on the third repeated listening situation.

If the sentence was not written down as it occurred originally on the testing cards, no credit was given, except in rare cases where such words as "in" might have been substituted for "into" or the like; in such cases where the meaning was accurate, full credit was given. The resulting scores on the sentence lists were in terms of 100 per cent. Ten sentences were included in each list. The maximum intelligibility score for each criteria was 100 per cent.

PHONETIC TRANSCRIPTION OF RECORDED MATERIAL

Phonetic analysis.—The 150 sentences and 750 PB words were phonetically analyzed to determine the possible number of errors for each sound and error category.

Error analysis.—Three individuals trained in phonetic transcription transcribed the recorded responses of the 150 sentences and 750 PB words spoken by the fifteen laryngectomized individuals. A comparison was made of the results of the three recorders. There was 96.4 per cent agreement. For the errors involved in the 3.6 per cent disagreement there were always two recorders who agreed.

The transcription of the recorded materials was then compared with the phonetic analysis of the original 150 sentences and 750 PB words. The errors were then classified.

ERROR CLASSIFICATION

The errors were classified in two ways:

1. The classification system employed by Anderson (1).
   a. The errors were categorized into consonants and vowels.
      1) Vowels— (i), (ɪ), (e), (ɛ), (æ), (ɑ), (o), (ɔ), (ʒ), (ʌ), (u), (ʊ), (ɑɪ), (ɑʊ).
      2) Consonants— (m), (n), (p), (b), (t), (f), (k), (g), (r), (l), (v), (θ), (ð), (h), (w), (j), (s), (ʃ), (tʃ), (dʒ), (d).
   b. The consonants were then classified further as:
      1) Voiced— (m), (n), (b), (d), (g), (r), (l), (v), (w), (dʒ), (ð), (j).
      2) Voiceless— (p), (t), (k), (f), (θ), (t), (h), (ʃ).
      3) Nasals— (m), (n).
      4) Stop-plosives— (p), (b), (t), (d), (k), (g), (t), (d).
      5) Semi-vowels— (r), (l).
      6) Fricatives— (f), (v), (θ), (s), (ʃ), (h), (ð).
      7) Glides— (w), (j).

The classification employed by Hyman (29) was similar to Anderson's with the following exceptions:

a. The sounds [r] and [l] were classified as glides rather than semi-vowels;

b. [tʃ] and [dʒ] as affricatives rather than fricatives.

2. The second classification system which permitted analysis of not only the categories of errors, but also the types, was derived by Hudgins and Numbers (27) and was employed in this study. They classified the errors as:

a. Consonant errors
   1) Surd-sonant
   2) Substitution
   3) Nasality
   4) Compound consonant
   5) Abutting consonant
   6) Arresting consonant
   7) Releasing consonant
b. Vowel errors
   1) Substitution
   2) Diphthongs

3) Diphthongization
4) Neutralization
5) Nasalization

In the preliminary transcription procedures as the transcribers collected and set up the error categories and types, it was apparent that all of Hudgins' and Numbers' error classifications utilized for the deaf did not apply to laryngectomized speakers. Other categories were found necessary and, therefore, were formulated; for the consonants, constructive compound; for the vowels, omission and constructive release. The following error categories were those used in the present investigation.

Consonant errors:

1. Errors involving the confusion of the surd-sonant (voice breath) distinction. This type of error occurs when [p] is given for [b], [t] for [d], [k] for [g], or [f] for [v], and [ch] for [j]; in other cases the reverse occurs, thus [b] may be given for [p]. This type of error may be completely confusing when the error produces a word with a totally different meaning such as hat for had, curl for girl, coat for goat.

2. Substitution of one consonant for another, such as [w] for [r], [t] for [s]; thus won is heard as run. Any consonant may conceivably be substituted for another.

3. Errors involving the articulation of compound consonants. These take one of two forms: (a) One or more of the members making up the compound may be dropped; thus street becomes st'eet, treet, or even teet; place becomes p'ace. (b) The members of the compound are given too much time and spoken too slowly with the result that adventitious syllables are added to the word; thus snow becomes su now, birds becomes bir dus, six becomes sikus. This type of error involves both the phonetic structure and the rhythmic patterns of the phrase.

4. Non-function of the arresting (final) consonant. The consonant movement is either dropped out entirely or the movement is incomplete, or again it may be so slow that its dynamic effect upon the preceding vowel is lost. In either case the syllable is not arrested and the vowel trails off slowly. Thus Paul becomes pau' . . ., house becomes hou' . . . .

5. Non-function of the releasing (initial) consonant. The consonant movement fails to close or to make the proper juncture with the opposing surface thus preventing a sufficient constriction for the air pressure to produce the consonantal effect upon the syllable. The articulatory movements may be made but they are too slow, or the proper closure is not made. They have no resemblance to the consonant movement; and becomes passive 'oral gestures' lacking in all the dynamic qualities of true consonants. The acoustic effect is that of dropping the consonant. (27), pp. 304-305.

6. Constructive compound—this error involves the introduction of an extraneous consonant with the original consonant of a syllable, the consonant movement; thus, fusing the two consonants into a compound consonant. Therefore, "lean" becomes "tlean," "last" becomes "blast."

Vowel errors:

1. Substitution of one vowel for another, thus paple for people, Jane for John.
2. Diphthongization of pure vowels. The slowing down of articulatory movements and a continuation of the voice during the transition from one sound to another often has the effect of making diphthongs out of pure vowels. For example, in the phrase 'how do you do' the vowels [oo] are continued while the articulatory movements are slowly moving to form the next consonant and the phrase becomes 'how-ee do-ee you-ee do.'
3. Neutralization of pure vowels. In this case the oral movements required for producing the vowel are not given full value and the vowel appears to fade out, loses its quality and becomes more like the neutral vowel -u-. The syllables are usually shortened and are not given their proper degree of stress. (27), pp. 306.
4. Omission—this error is the complete dropping of the pure vowel.
5. Constructive release—this error involves the introduction of an extraneous releasing consonant. Thus "are" becomes "tare," "only" becomes "bonely," "age" becomes "dage."

This type of analysis appeared desirable in the evaluation of the articulatory errors and their effect on intelligibility of laryngectomized speakers. Furthermore, the auditors' written responses of the recorded materials were evaluated to estimate the effects of different articulatory errors on speech intelligibility.

PROCEDURES IN CHECKING SPEECH RHYTHM

Since it is known that articulatory precision is positively correlated with speech rhythm (word accent and grouping) it was considered desirable to investigate the speech rhythm used by laryngectomized subjects in speaking the sentences. Three members of the American Speech and Hearing Association with advanced certification in speech first independently determined and wrote down what they believed to be the normal rhythm of the sentences. The rhythm patterns were further substantiated after the sentences were read aloud by each member. After the recordings were evaluated a comparison of the patterns revealed a

98 per cent agreement. For the sentences involved in the 2 per cent dis-agreement there were always two recorders who agreed. Utilizing the established "normal" rhythm pattern the three recorders listened and wrote down independently their evaluations of the speech rhythm employed by each laryngectomized person speaking a group of ten different unrelated sentences. Rhythm was recorded as being "normal," "non-rhythmic," or "abnormal." These terms are to be understood as defined by Hudgins and Numbers:

> *Normal rhythm* included all those in which the accents were properly placed, in which the normal English grouping of syllables obtained, and in which the rate of syllable utterance was such that grouping was possible.
>
> The rhythm . . . was classified as *abnormal* when the rhythmic pattern conflicted with, or did not conform to a normal English pattern for that sentence. . . .
>
> Sentences were classified as non-rhythmic when there was a complete absence of grouping, when each syllable in the phrase was spoken slowly and with the same degree of stress, and as a single breath group. . . . (27), p. 352.

The three judges agreed in their evaluation on 96 per cent of the sentences; for the remaining 4 per cent at least two judges agreed.

The relative effect of rhythmic errors upon speech intelligibility was then studied in relation to the errors of the auditors on the recorded sentences.

SURGICAL INFORMATION

Since the literature has indicated that various laryngologists have been concerned with the amount of tissue removed during surgery for laryngectomy, it was thought profitable to investigate this aspect for the laryngectomized speakers in this study. A surgery report data sheet (see Appendix) was prepared with the help and guidance of the late Dr. Blaisdell. The cooperating surgeons who performed the laryngec-tomies supplied the essential information for each subject.

HISTORY INFORMATION

History information was obtained from the laryngectomized subjects in this study through means of a questionnaire procedure. A question-naire was prepared (see Appendix) consisting of thirty-seven questions relating to the following areas:

1. speech training prior to surgery;
2. types of communication after surgery;
3. types of training received and by whom;

4. ability (since surgery) to lift weights, sneeze, smell and taste;
5. presence of discomfort, pain or fatigue since surgery;
6. presence of hoarseness, pain, coughing, loss of voice before surgery;
7. extent of recreational activities before and after surgery;
8. adjustment to handicap.

Items for the questionnaire were suggested by the literature reviewed, cooperating laryngologists and the laryngectomized subjects. The nature of the questions was discussed with each subject on his initial orientation. They were then permitted to write their replies to the questions at the Center, or if conditions prevented their completing them at that time, they completed them at home. Clarification was requested in cases of ambiguous replies.

CINEFLUOROGRAPHIC FILM VIEWS

Cinefluorographic film views were taken of ten laryngectomized subjects (five high and five low in intelligibility) and one normal subject. The film views were completed through the cooperation of and under the direction of Drs. Watson, Ramsey and Graniak of the Rochester Medical School. The equipment consisted of a 35 millimeter camera with a Kodak 110-mm Fluro Ektar $f/0.75$ lens and a synchronization apparatus. In addition a Dupont Patterson E-2 fluoroscopic screen and Kodak Lenograph ortho film, 35-mm (green sensitive) were employed. The X-ray generator employed was the KX-1 and the X-ray tube was a CRT 1-2. The exposure was 15 r for all individuals. A more detailed description of the equipment and procedures is provided by Watson and Weinberg (64).

Two views were taken for each speaker:
1. lateral, exposing the head, neck and esophageal areas;
2. frontal, exposing the rib cage and diaphragm areas.

The subjects spoke the same passage of thirty syllables (which was tape recorded). This tape recorded material was synchronized with the original film.

CHAPTER FOUR

RESULTS AND DISCUSSION

SILENT BREATHING COORDINATIONS

KYMOGRAPH TRACINGS WERE MADE IN SILENT BREATH-ing for both the normal and laryngectomized groups. Previous research by Stetson (50) and others has established the silent and speech breathing coordinations for normal subjects. There is no reason to believe that the normal subjects of this study differ significantly in breathing coordinations from the established findings. The interest here is in discovering if there are any significant differences between the normal group and the laryngectomized group in silent breathing.

Figure 8 represents a kymograph tracing of two laryngectomized subjects during one minute of silent breathing. Speaker M. O. G., in I, reveals five regular, normal breathing cycles. Speaker II, A. L., presents tracings showing six complete cycles. The silent breathing coordinations for both these normal speakers indicate clear, complete excursions of the chest and abdominal walls with unequivocal demarcations between each cycle. The laryngectomized subjects' tracings are III and IV. Speaker P. S. in tracing III has not quite completed seven cycles, while speaker G. B. in tracing IV has not quite completed six cycles. For these speakers, as for the normals, the cycles are clearly marked and differentiated. The tracings reveal a marked similarity in the breathing coordinations between the normal and the laryngectomized speakers.

Table 1 summarizes the data for one minute of silent breathing for the normal and for the laryngectomized groups. The measurements taken during silent breathing include: (1) cycles per minute; (2) abdominal, chest and combined amplitudes, measured in millimeters. The differences between the means of the group of laryngectomized individuals and the normal group reveal the laryngectomized speakers to have a greater number of breathing cycles per minute and greater abdominal, chest and combined mean amplitude.

The normal group has a mean of 16.47 in cycles per minute while the laryngectomized speakers have a mean of 19.27 cycles. Although this

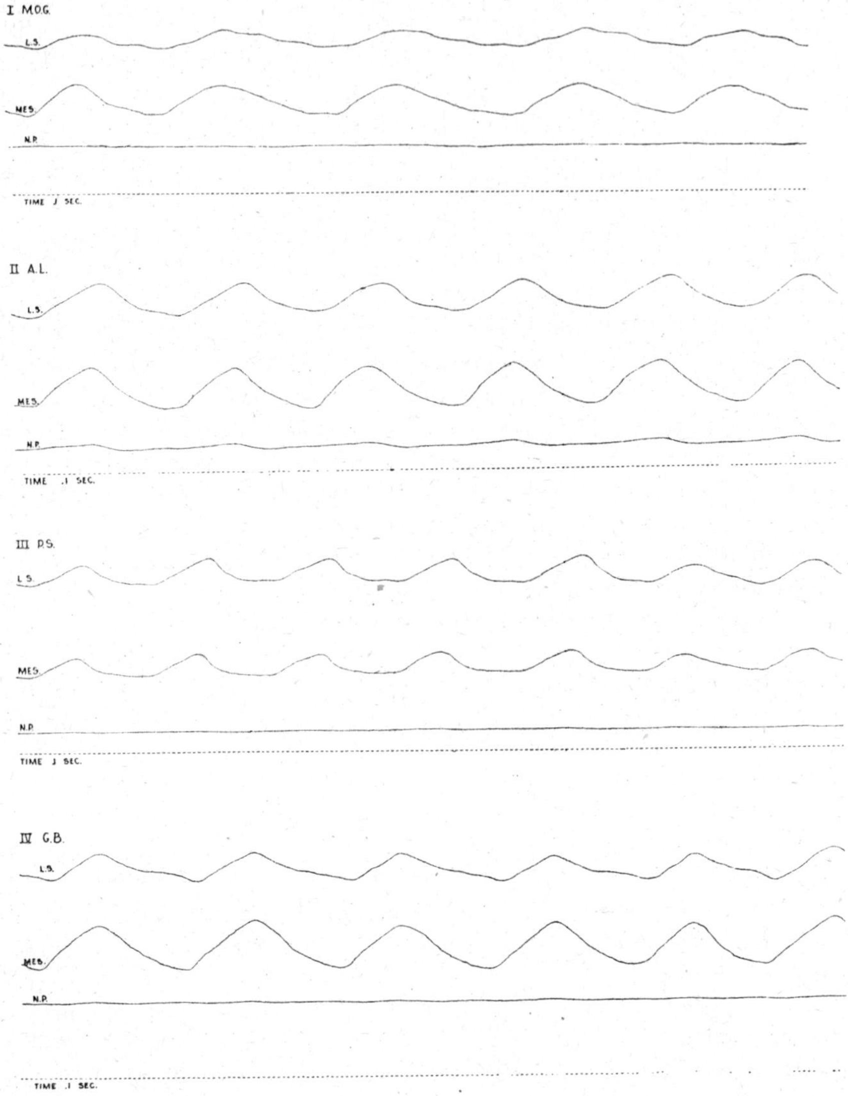

FIG. 8. Kymograms of one-minute duration of silent breathing of two normal speakers and two laryngectomized speakers.

1. *Subject:* M.O.G.—Normal speaker.

    L.S.   Tracing of the movement of the chest wall, taken at the lower sternum during silent breathing. The form is regular and smooth.

    Mes.   Tracing of the movement of the abdominal wall at the mesogastric level during silent breathing. The form is regular and the cycles are equal in number and synchronous with the movement of the chest wall.

Fig. 8.—*Continued*

N.P. Tracing of the syllable pulse taken at the epigastric level. There are no syllable pulses in silent breathing. The tracing is a straight line.

II. *Subject:* A.L.—Normal speaker.

L.S. Tracing of the movement of the chest wall, taken at the lower sternum during silent breathing. The form is regular and smooth.

Mes. Tracing of the movement of the abdominal wall at the mesogastric level during silent breathing. The amplitude of the movement of the abdominal wall is slightly greater than the chest.

N.P. Tracing of the syllable pulse taken at the epigastric level. There are no syllable pulses, but there are slight breaks in the line due to equipment adjustments.

III. *Subject:* P.S.—Laryngectomized speaker.

L.S. Tracing of the movement of the chest wall, taken at the lower sternum during silent breathing. The form is regular and smooth.

Mes. Tracing of the movement of the abdominal wall at the mesogastric level during silent breathing. The cycles are regular and smooth.

N.P. Tracing of the syllable pulse taken at the epigastric level. There are no syllable pulses.

IV. *Subject:* G.B.—Laryngectomized speaker.

L.S. Tracing of the movement of the chest wall, taken at the lower sternum during silent breathing. The form is regular and smooth.

Mes. Tracing of the movement of the abdominal wall at the mesogastric level during silent breathing. The amplitude of the movement of the abdominal wall is slightly greater than the chest.

N.P. Tracing of the syllable pulse taken at the epigastric level. There are no syllable pulses.

There is great similarity of the kymogram tracings for the four speakers. Time is recorded in .1 seconds.

TABLE 1

MEANS, VARIANCES, STANDARD DEVIATIONS, DIFFERENCES BETWEEN THE MEANS, t AND F VALUES FOR ONE MINUTE OF SILENT BREATHING OF THE NORMAL AND LARYNGECTOMIZED SPEAKERS, FOR CYCLES PER MINUTE, AND FOR ABDOMINAL, CHEST, AND COMBINED AMPLITUDES IN MILLIMETERS

Variables	Normal N = 15			Laryngectomized N = 15			$\overline{X}_{lar.}\overline{X}_{n.}$	t	F
	$\overline{X}_{n.}$	σ^2	σ	$\overline{X}_{lar.}$	σ^2	σ			
Cycles per minute	16.47	6.98	2.64	19.27	15.35	3.92	2.80	2.30*	2.20
Abdominal	10.93	20.12	4.49	13.32	20.85	4.57	2.39	1.45	1.04
Chest	12.42	14.12	3.76	17.12	48.99	7.00	4.70	2.29ˣ	3.47*
Combined	11.68	11.99	3.46	15.25	21.15	4.60	3.57	2.40*	1.76

n. = Normal speakers
lar. = Laryngectomized speakers

xx = .01 Indicates significance
x = .05 of t when F is significant

Combined amplitude - Mean of the chest and abdominal amplitudes

df = 28
t.01 = 2.763
t.02 = 2.467
t.05 = 2.048
df = 14
t.01 = 2.977
t.02 = 2.624
t.05 = 2.145
** = .01
* = .05

F df = 14 and 14
F.02 = 3.70
F.05 = 3.34
F (Interpolated)
.10 = 2.48

difference of 2.80 cycles is significant at the .05 level of confidence, never-theless both of the means fall within the normal range, which has been quoted by others as being between 12 and 20 cycles per minute (16).

The mean chest amplitude for the normal speakers in the present study is 12.42 millimeters; for the laryngectomized speakers the mean is 17.12 millimeters. The difference of 4.70 millimeters is significant at the .05 level of confidence with a t value of 2.29 and an F value of 3.47, which is significant at the .05 level.[1] The combined mean amplitude difference between the mean of the two groups proves to be significant at the .05 level with a t value of 2.40. The t value of 2.39 for the differ-ence between the means of the abdominal amplitudes of the two groups does not prove to be significant.

Although the two groups are shown to be significantly different in relation to number of cycles per minute and chest amplitude, a con-sideration of Figures 8 and 9 reveals marked similarity between the groups. Figure 9 shows a distribution of the number of breathing cycles

[1]In all situations where the assumption of homogeneity of variance, essential to the t test is not met, the t table is is entered with 14 df. instead of 28 df. This will be maintained throughout the study (13).

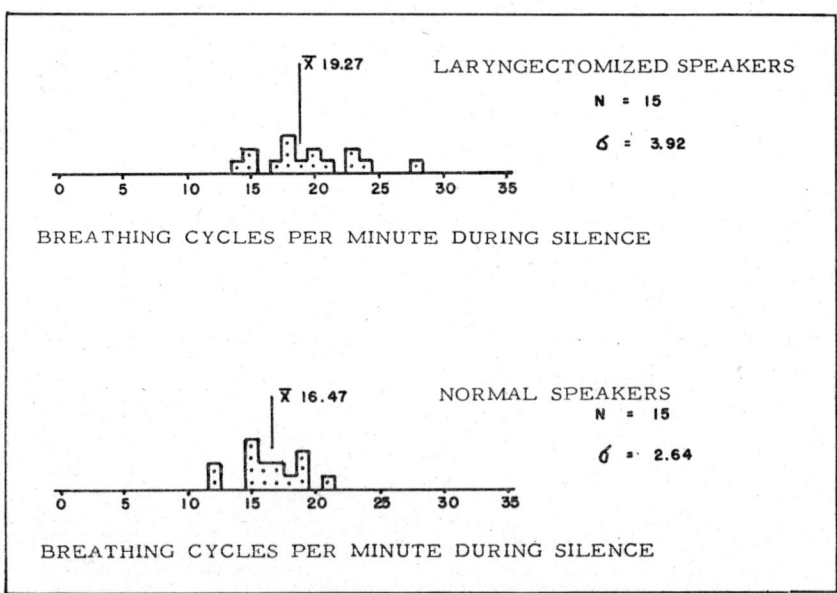

FIG. 9. Distribution of breathing cycles per minute during silence for the laryngectomized speakers and the normal speakers, showing x̄, N, and σ for both groups.

per minute during silence for normal and laryngectomized subjects. This figure also reveals similarity in means and variability.

Figure 10 represents scattergrams of the abdominal and chest amplitudes in millimeters during silent breathing for the normal and the laryngectomized speakers. The zero difference lines are included in these diagrams. The individuals whose values fall on the zero difference line have equal amplitude for the chest and the abdomen. Those whose values fall below this line show greater abdominal amplitude, and those who fall above the line display greater chest amplitude. There are four normal speakers who have greater abdominal amplitude, and, likewise, four laryngectomized speakers who have greater abdominal amplitude as compared to their chest amplitude.

The differences indicated in chest amplitude and cycles per minute, which are statistically significant, need not necessarily be clinically meaningful for the following reasons:

1. The configuration patterns of the kymograms in Figure 8 indicate similar, smooth, differentiated cycles for both groups.
2. The mean number of breathing cycles per minute for the laryngectomized group falls within the normal range. (Ten of the fifteen laryngectomized speakers fall within this range.)
3. The laryngectomized speakers' greatest number of breathing cycles (2.80) over a minute's duration of silent breathing is not likely to be clinically meaningful.
4. There is less resistance to the moving air columns and thus greater escape of air.
5. Greater escape of air and the decreased length of air passageway facilitate the accumulation of carbon dioxide which necessitates a greater number of respiratory cycles.
6. In reference to the significant difference in chest amplitude, the cooperating laryngologists in this study found, clinically, that laryngectomized individuals increased in chest expansion several inches during the first post-operative year.
7. The variability of the normal group and that of the laryngectomized group in cycles per minute are similar.

SPEECH BREATHING

The kymograph recordings in speech breathing were examined for any significant differences which might exist between the normal speakers and the laryngectomized speakers. It was hypothesized by Stetson (57) that the speech breathing coordinations of laryngectomized

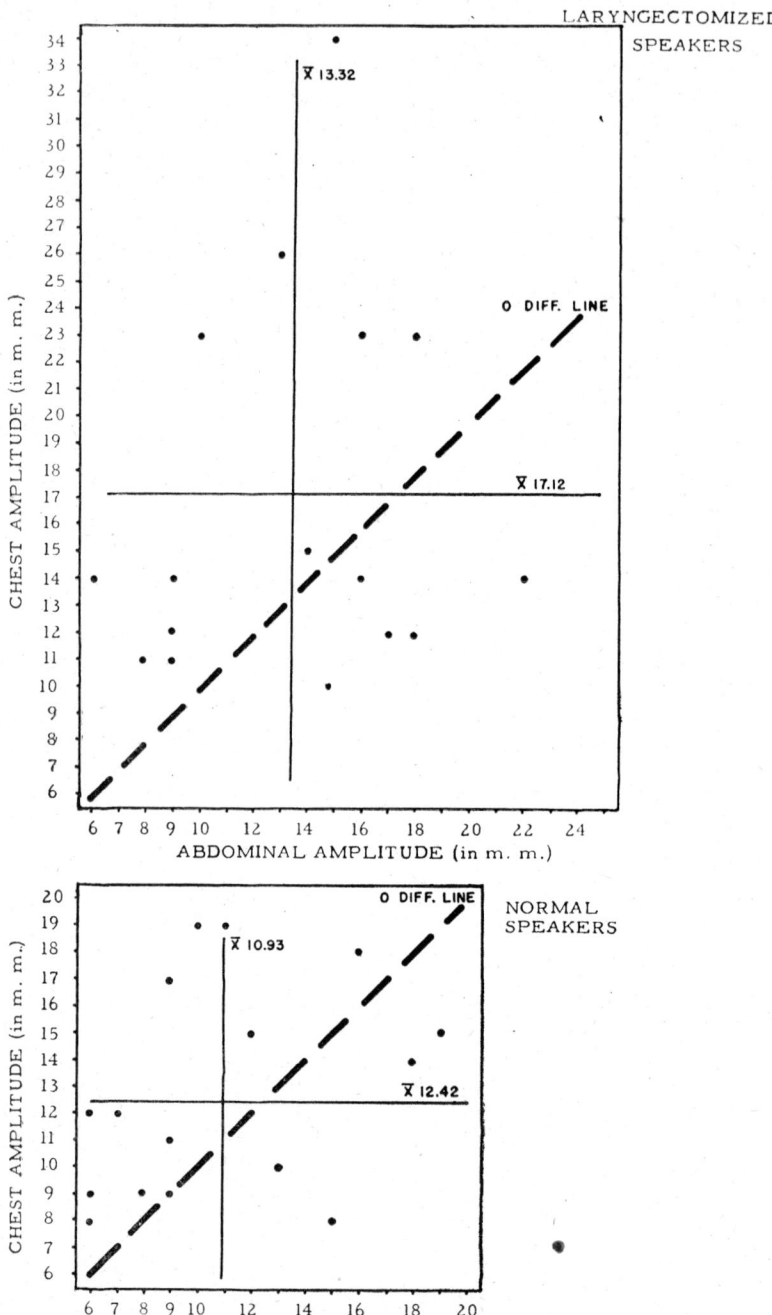

FIG. 10. Scatter diagrams for the normal and laryngectomized speakers for chest and abdominal amplitudes in millimeters during silent breathing, indicating means and zero difference lines for both groups.

speakers were those of the normal speakers. An inspection of the kymograph tracings of the sixty-syllable paragraph for the normal and laryngectomized groups revealed certain similarities but also specific differences.

Figure 11 represents the kymograph tracings of two normal and two laryngectomized speakers. The first two normal speakers, A. L. and D. C., in tracings I and II, completed the sixty-syllable paragraph in four phrases, while the laryngectomized speaker, H. G., in tracing III, spoke the paragraph in nine phrases, only five of which are represented in the tracing presented. Speaker F. M., in tracing IV, also a laryngectomized speaker, used thirty-five phrases in speaking the paragraph, fifteen of which are shown in the tracing. The tracings of H. G., while showing a greater number of phrases, bear a marked similarity to the coordinations of the two normal speakers. Speaker F. M. used many more phrases, but each phrase was distinct and the syllable pulses below indicated that he was using one or two syllables per phrase. These two laryngectomized speakers were judged to be among the more intelligible of the laryngectomized group.

Figure 12 represents four laryngectomized speakers who were judged to be low in intelligibility. Speaker R. C. M., in tracing I, revealed marked deviations from the normal tracings. The tracing at the lower sternum, representing the thoracic movement in speech, and the tracing at the mesogastric area, representing the abdominal movement in speech, were consistently out of phase. The action of the chest walls was not regular and represented changing movement, while the action of the abdominal wall indicated a different number of cycles and also out-of-phase coordinations. The negative pressure tracing (N. P.) appeared to be consistent with the chest wall and seemed to follow with a short delay the action of the abdominal wall.

Speaker M. A., tracing II, in Figure 12, though using a greater number of phrases and differences in amplitude, still showed indications of the in-phase movements of the chest and abdominal walls. Excessive pressure was used at some points and a minimum of pressure was used at other points. The negative pressure stylus appeared to be in contraphase with the stylus of the mesogastric area.

The tracings of speaker G. B. in tracing III, indicate the same type of coordinations as speaker M. A., with the additional abdominal out-of-phase movements at certain points. The negative pressure line for the syllable pulse indicates that this speaker was using one syllable for each phrase.

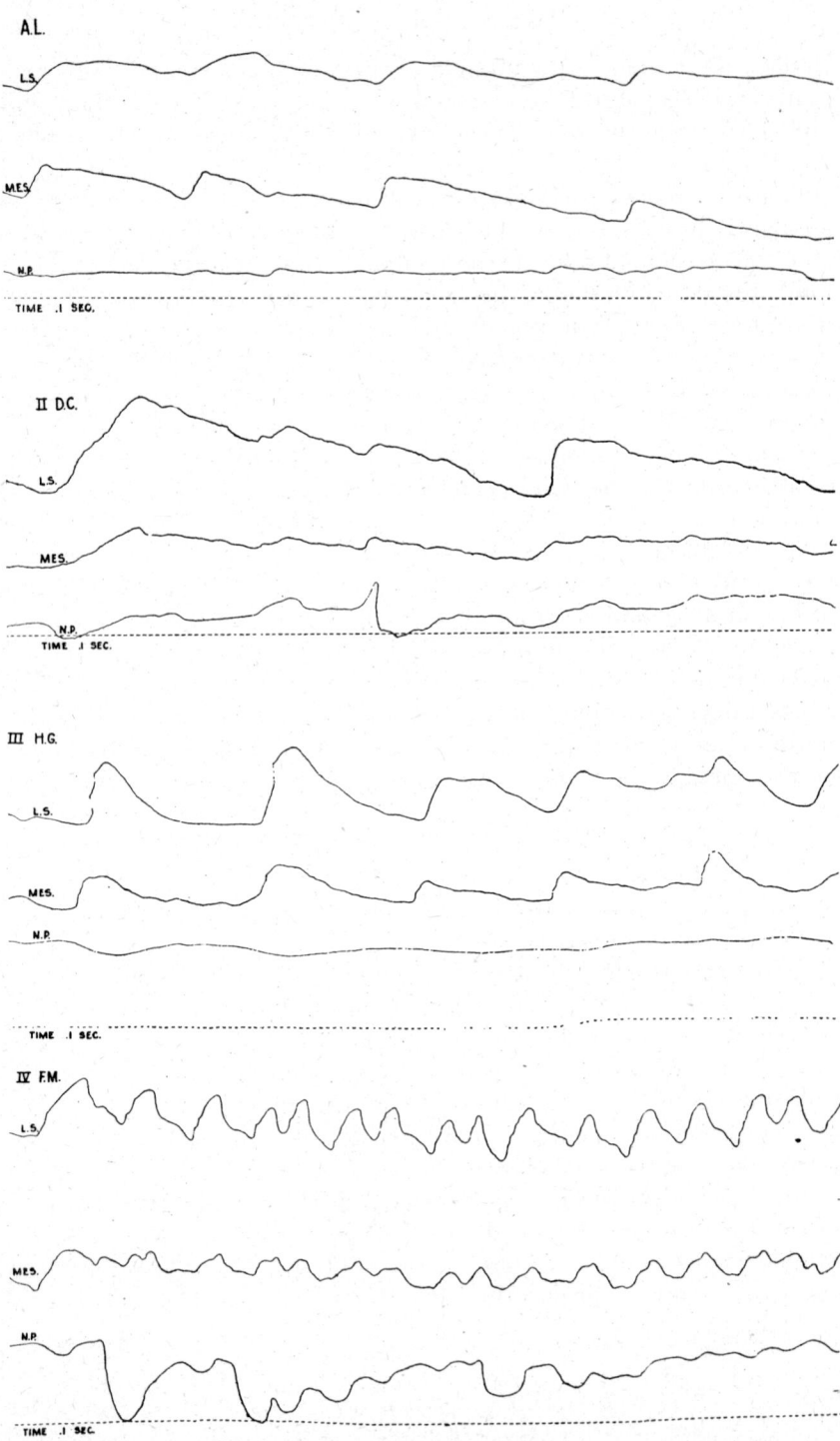

FIG. 11.

Fig. 11. Kymograms of the sixty-syllable paragraph spoken by two normal subjects and two laryngectomized subjects.

I. *Subject:* A.L.—Normal speaker.

   L.S.   Tracing of the movement of the chest wall, taken at the lower sternum. The configuration of the phrasing movement is clear. There are four distinct phrase excursions.

   Mes.   Tracing of the movement of the abdominal wall at the mesogastric level. The phrase movements are distinct and in phase with the movements of the chest wall. The demarcation between phrases is clear cut.

   N.P.   Tracing of the syllable pulse taken at the epigastric level. The syllables are grouped in rhythmical feet.

II. *Subject:* D.C.—Normal speaker.

   L.S.   Tracing of the movement of the chest wall, taken at the lower sternum. Greater chest action is indicated by the large amplitude. The speaker uses four phrases for the sixty-syllable paragraph.

   Mes.   Tracing of the movement of the abdominal wall at the mesogastric level. There is less abdominal action but movements are in phase.

   N.P.   Tracing of the syllable pulse taken at the epigastric level. The grouping of syllables in feet is clearly indicated by the regular sharp rises and depressions in the tracing.

III. *Subject:* H.G.—Laryngectomized speaker (High intelligibility).

   L.S.   Tracing of the movement of the chest wall, taken at the lower sternum. The clear-cut phrase movements executed by the chest wall are readily observable. Notice the slightly greater chest amplitude indicating greater chest excursion.

   Mes.   Tracing of the movement of the abdominal wall at the mesogastric level. The speaker uses well-defined phrasing movements, clearly indicating that the abdominal and chest walls are in phase.

   N.P.   Tracing of the syllable pulse taken at the epigastric level. While the tracings are not strongly indicated, nevertheless there is a rise within each syllable revealing the rhythm pattern of the syllables in a well-defined phrase movement. Note the similarity of configuration for the above three speakers.

IV. *Subject:* F.M.—Laryngectomized speaker (High intelligibility).

   L.S.   Tracing of the movement of the chest wall, taken at the lower sternum. While there is a greater number of movements, they are regular and somewhat smooth. The greater number of movements indicates that the speaker uses a greater number of phrases in speaking the sixty-syllable paragraph.

   Mes.   Tracing of the movement of the abdominal wall at the mesogastric level. Note the clear-cut demarcation and consistent synchrony of the chest and abdominal wall movements. The greater amplitude of the chest would indicate greater excursion of the chest walls, but the movements are in phase and regular.

   N.P.   Tracing of the syllable pulse taken at the epigastric level. With the exception of the first two syllables, each syllable receives practically the same stress. The speech is non-rhythmical but intelligible, since the movements are well-defined and synchronous. Each phrase contains one syllable, but there are no exaggerated time intervals between utterances.

Time is recorded in .1 seconds.

Speaker J. K., in tracing IV, appeared to have good chest wall movement, but inadequate abdominal wall movement, with out-of-phase coordinations at different points in the tracings.

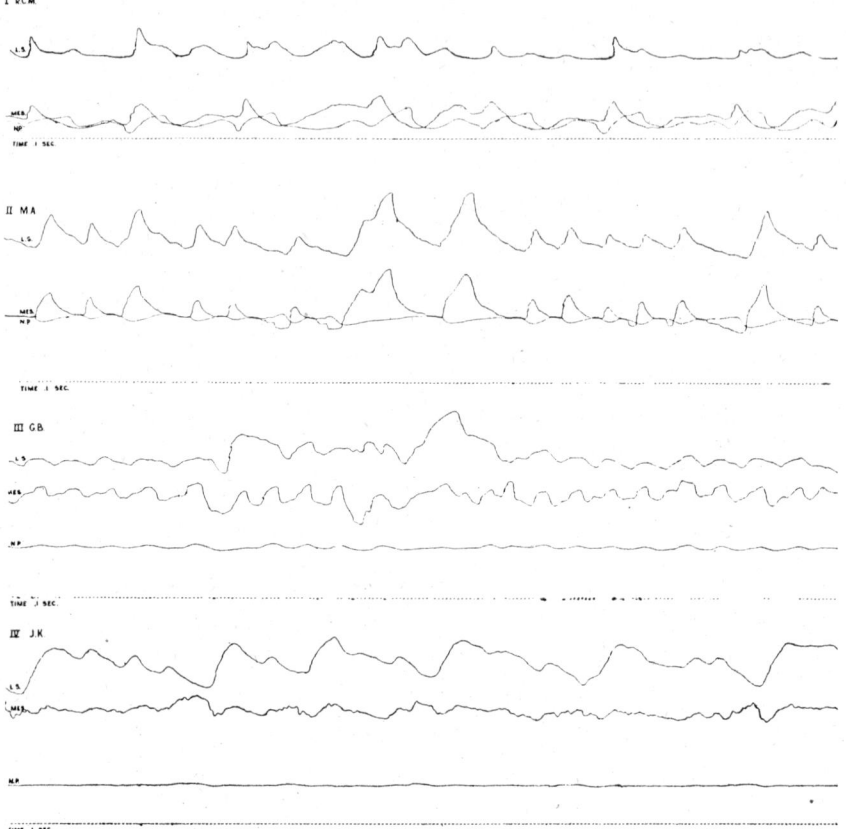

FIG. 12. Kymograms of the sixty-syllable paragraph spoken by four laryngectomized speakers.

I. *Subject:* R.C.M.—Laryngectomized speaker (Low intelligibility).

L.S.   Tracing of the movement of the chest wall, taken at the lower sternum. The amplitude of the movements is variable, indicating excessive amounts of breath used at certain places, while there is a lack of breath pressure at other places during the speaking process. Notice the greater number of phrases appearing at the beginning of the tracing, and the fewer phrases at the end of the tracing, indicating diminution of breath. Tracings would indicate abnormal rhythm.

Mes.   Tracing of the movement of the abdominal wall at the mesogastric level. Notice the opposite phase movements frequently occurring throughout the tracing, indicating an outward movement of the chest wall and a simultaneous inward movement of the abdominal wall, indicating the two are out of phase.

N.P   Tracing of the syllable pulse taken at the epigastric level. The individual syllable pulses are clearly shown, revealing abnormal groupings and inclusion of extra syllable movements. The entire speech-breathing process is out of phase and disynchronous.

Fig. 12.—*Continued*

II. *Subject:* M.A.—Laryngectomized speaker (Low intelligibility).

L.S. Tracing of the movement of the chest wall, taken at the lower sternum. Note the variance of the amplitude excessively high in phrases 3, 7, 8 and 14, indicating the excessive amount of breath used for the phrases at these junctures.

Mes. Tracing of the movement of the abdominal wall at the mesogastric level. Note the similarity of the configurations between chest and abdominal movements. Also note the exaggerated movements indicating the use of high pressures.

N.P. Tracing of the syllable pulse taken at the epigastric level. There is one pulse with each phrase, but there is a difference in pressures, revealing abnormal rhythm.

III. *Subject:* G.B.—Laryngectomized speaker (Low intelligibility).

L.S. Tracing of the movement of the chest wall, taken at the lower sternum. Note in irregularity and variance of amplitudes and greater number of movements in the tracings. These factors would indicate excessive expenditure of breath. The greater number of phrases comprising one or two syllables each are indicated by the tracing N.P.

Mes. Tracing of the movement of the abdominal wall at the mesogastric level. Note the irregularity and the greater number of movements. Compared with the chest movements, there appears to be greater irregularity. Note also extra movements and out-of-phase relationships indicated by the outward movement of the chest walls and inward movement of the abdominal walls. The chest and abdominal movements are disynchronous at certain places.

N.P. Tracing of the syllable pulse taken at the epigastric level. Each syllable appears to coincide with the phrase movement in the mesogastric tracing. Each syllable appears to receive the same stress, but variance in chest and abdominal amplitudes indicate abnormal rhythm.

IV. *Subject:* J.K.—Laryngectomized speaker (Low intelligibility).

L.S. Tracing the movement of the chest wall, taken at the lower sternum. Tracing reflects regular movement, but excessive amplitude. This would indicate excessive amount of breath used for the phrase.

Mes. Tracing of the movement of the abdominal wall at the mesogastric level. Tracing indicates diminished movement of the abdominal wall and also irregularity of movement. The chest and abdominal walls indicate disynchrony at certain stages in the speech process.

N.P. Tracing of the syllable pulse taken at the epigastric level. Tracings show diminished syllable pulses, indicating that most of the effort for speaking puts the chest under high pressure.

Time is recorded in .1 seconds.

Table 2 summarizes the findings for the normal and the laryngectomized groups in speaking the sixty-syllable paragraph. It is noted that the laryngectomized group took more time in speaking the paragraph and used a greater number of phrases. They also used greater time per phrase and had fewer number of syllables per phrase than the normal group. The two variables, time per phrase and number of syllables, are included for comparative purposes. Analysis of these in the study have not contributed greatly since the ratio of the two variables appears to cancel out the differences found within each. In

TABLE 2

MEANS, VARIANCES, STANDARD DEVIATIONS, DIFFERENCES BETWEEN MEANS, t AND F VALUES
FOR SPEECH BREATHING OF THE NORMAL AND LARYNGECTOMIZED SPEAKERS, ON THE SIXTY-
SYLLABLE PARAGRAPH, FOR TIME, NUMBER OF PHRASES, TIME PER PHRASE,
NUMBER OF SYLLABLES PER PHRASE; AND FOR ABDOMINAL, CHEST,
AND COMBINED AMPLITUDES IN MILLIMETERS

Variables	Normal N = 15			Laryngectomized N = 15			$\bar{X}_{lar.} \cdot \bar{X}_{n.}$	t	F
	$\bar{X}_{n.}$	σ^2	σ	$\bar{X}_{lar.}$	σ^2	σ			
Time	19.14	7.42	2.72	43.81	861.88	29.35	24.67	3.24^{xx}	115.67**
No. of phrases	5.20	2.60	1.61	27.40	261.69	16.17	22.20	5.29^{xx}	100.65**
Time per phrase	3.92	1.08	1.03	1.72	0.47	0.69	-2.20	6.85**	2.27
No. of syllables per phrase	12.52	12.70	3.57	3.12	4.21	2.05	-9.40	8.85**	3.02
Abdominal	9.93	13.50	3.67	9.49	13.05	3.61	-0.44	0.34	1.03
Chest	13.11	24.30	4.93	11.33	21.02	4.58	-1.78	1.04	1.16
Combined	11.52	11.00	3.32	10.41	8.50	2.92	-1.11	1.01	1.30

Amplitude (label spanning Abdominal, Chest, Combined rows)

n. = Normal speakers
lar. = Laryngectomized speakers

xx = .01   Indicates significance
x = .05   of t when F is significant

df = 28
t.01 = 2.763
t.02 = 2.467
t.05 = 2.048
df = 14
t.01 = 2.977
t.02 = 2.624
t.05 = 2.145
** = .01
* = .05

F df = 14 and 14
F.02 = 3.70
F.05 = 3.34
F(Interpolated)
F.10 = 2.48

reference to measured amplitude, the abdominal, chest and combined amplitudes are greater for the normal group than for the laryngectomized group.

The mean of 19.14 seconds in total speaking time for the normal group contrasts significantly with the mean of 43.81 seconds for the laryngectomized group. The diffence of 24.6 seconds, with a t value of 3.24, is significant at the .01 level of confidence. The variances of the two groups are also significantly different at the .02 level of confidence.

Figure 13 shows the distribution for the normal and laryngectomized speakers for total time in seconds in speaking the sixty-syllable paragraph. Each of the laryngectomized speakers is above the mean of the normal speakers in time taken to speak the paragraph. Ten laryngectomized speakers, although appearing above the normal mean, comprised a distribution of their own similar to the normals, while the remaining five laryngectomized individuals appearing above the mean were scattered over a sixty-second period of time. The normal group members all produced the paragraph in less than twenty-five seconds.

In number of phrases used in speaking the sixty-syllable paragraph, the two groups also differ greatly. The laryngectomized individuals with a mean number of phrases of 27.40 used over four times as many phrases for the speaking of the paragraph as did the normals with a

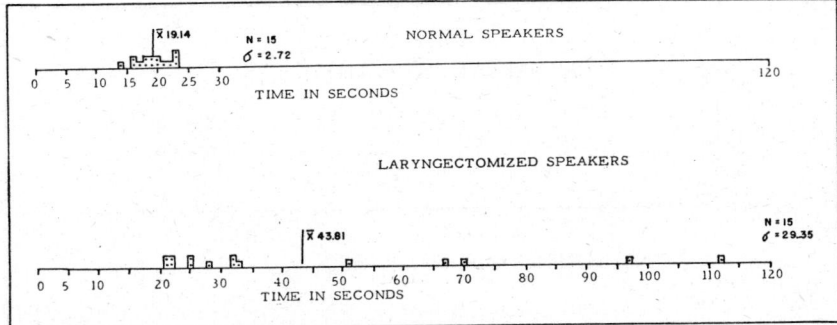

FIG. 13. Distribution of total time in seconds for the normal and laryngectomized subjects speaking the sixty-syllable paragraph, showing x̄, N, and σ
for each group.

mean of 5.20. The difference, resulting in a t of 5.29, is significant beyond
the .01 level of confidence. Figure 14 shows that all of the laryngectomized speakers fall above the mean of the normal speakers in number of
phrases used. Figure 14 is similar to Figure 13 in that five of the laryngectomized speakers form their own distribution above the mean for the
total group of laryngectomized speakers.

The two groups differ significantly also in time per phrase and in
number of syllables; the differences here are significant beyond the .01
level, with t values of 6.85 and 8.85 respectively.

The two groups do not differ significantly in the abdominal, chest
or combined mean amplitude measures. Figure 15 shows scattergrams
of the mean amplitudes of the chest and abdominal measures for the
normal and the laryngectomized speakers. When these diagrams are
compared with Figure 10, which represents the abdominal and chest
amplitudes in silence, interesting differences are noted. There were four
normal and four laryngectomized speakers who had greater abdominal
amplitude during silence. But, during speech, as seen in Figure 15, three
of the normal speakers had greater abdominal amplitude; one normal
speaker was one the zero difference line. In contrast, seven of the laryngectomized speakers were found to have greater abdominal amplitude.
The zero difference line separates the laryngectomized group into seven
with greater abdominal amplitude and eight with greater chest amplitude.

Kallen indicated that a clue to the location of the vicarious air
chamber and the pseudo-glottis was to be found in the extent of the
body wall movements. "The lower these two structures lie, the more

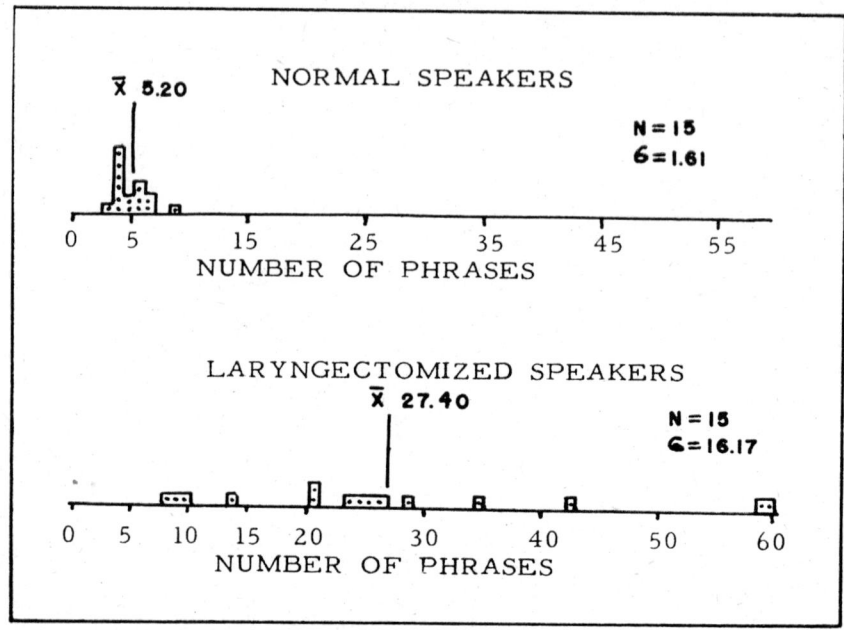

Fig. 14. Distribution of the number of phrases for the normal and laryngectomized subjects speaking the sixty-syllable paragraph, showing x̄, N, and σ
for each group.

marked the abdominal component of respiration is likely to be, and
the higher they lie, the more the thoracic element is likely to play a
part in the new way of speaking" (28, pp. 488-489). Anderson (1) in
his study substantiated this point of view.

Figure 16 illustrates the distributions for the abdominal, chest and
combined amplitudes for the normal and laryngectomized groups in
silence and in speech. The means between the normal and the laryngectomized groups for the amplitudes as measured during speech show
marked similarity. Although the mean amplitudes measured during
silence are not as comparable as during speech breathing, the similarities between silence and speech breathing are discernible.

COMPARISONS WITHIN THE NORMAL AND LARYNGECTOMIZED GROUPS FOR
ABDOMINAL, CHEST AND COMBINED AMPLITUDES IN SILENCE AND IN SPEECH

Tables 1 and 2 provide information concerning the differences
between the two groups. In reference to the amplitude variable during
silence, the laryngectomized speakers had significantly greater chest

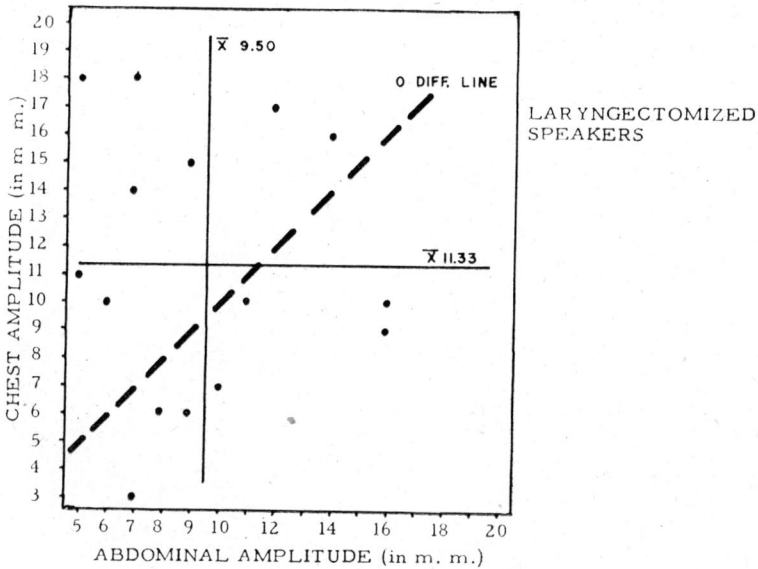

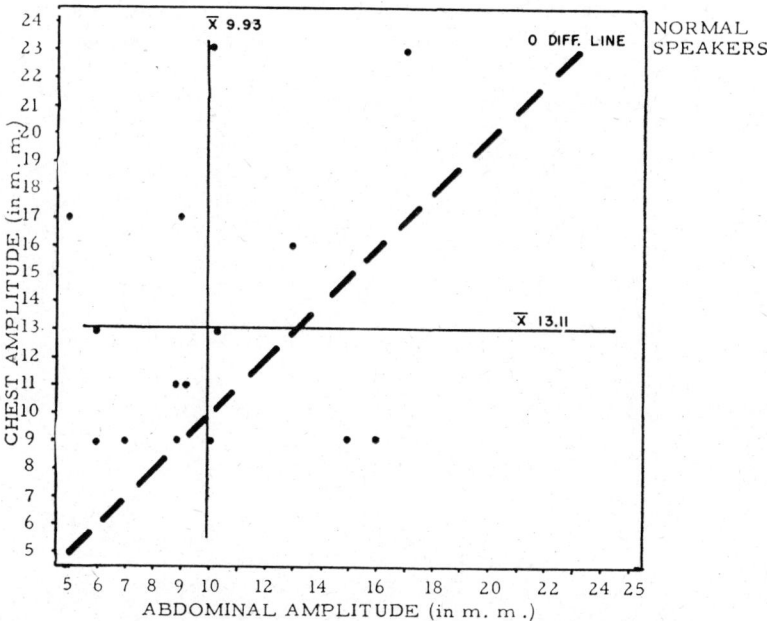

FIG. 15. Abdominal amplitude (in millimeters) and chest amplitude for normal and laryngectomized speakers during speech, with means and zero difference lines.

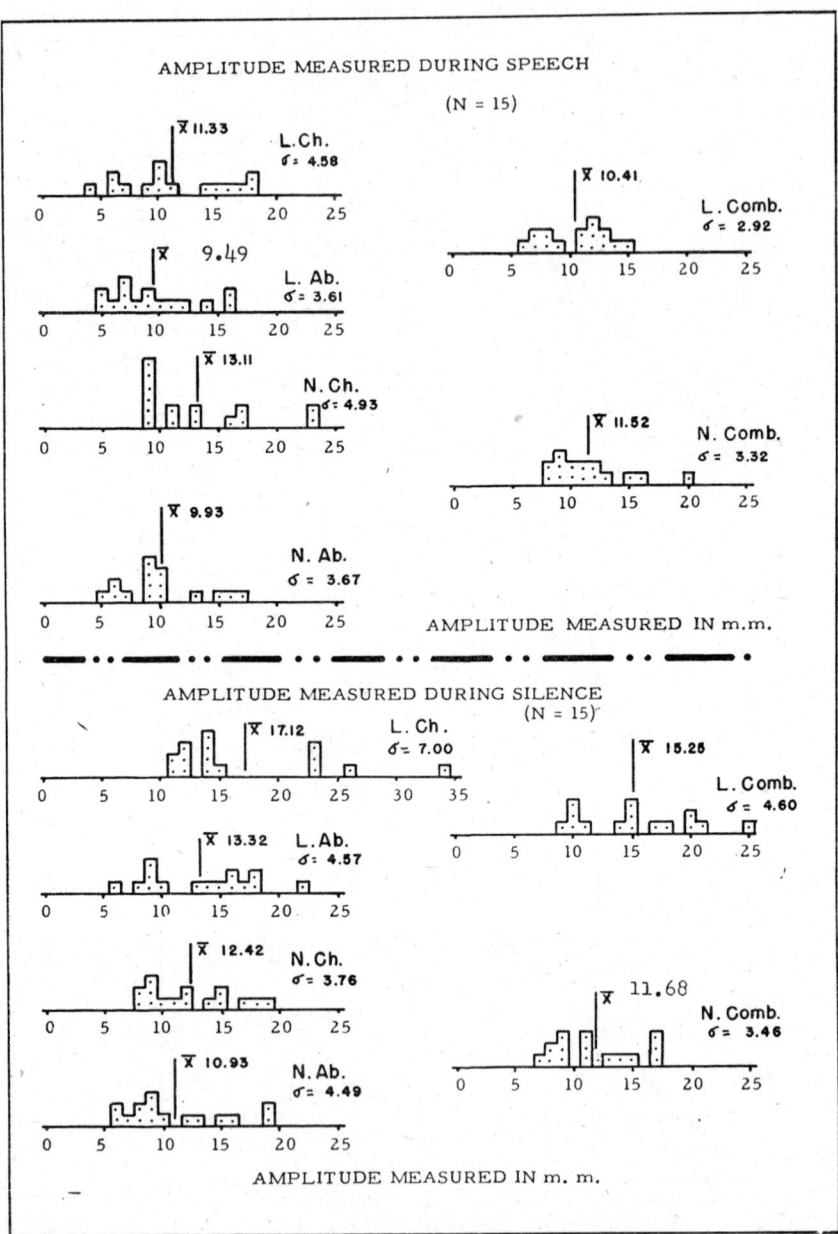

FIG. 16. Chest amplitude measured in millimeters with abdominal and combined amplitudes for normal and laryngectomized groups in silence and in speech.

amplitude than the normal speakers. The speech breathing amplitude results indicate no significant differences between groups. It was thought that it might be profitable to investigate the differences of these variables within the normal group and within the laryngectomized group in silence and in speech. In this instance, the null hypothesis being investigated is that the mean difference equals zero. No F test is necessary since only one group of differences was investigated. Table 3 summarizes the data in reference to this question and shows the mean differences (D) and the t scores. In the normal group no significant differences are found, although less chest amplitude and greater abdominal and combined amplitudes are shown in silence, as compared to speech.

The laryngectomized group shows means for the abdominal, chest and combined amplitudes during silence which are greater than the mean amplitudes during speech, and these mean differences are all

TABLE 3

MEANS, MEAN DIFFERENCE, AND t VALUES WITHIN THE NORMAL AND THE LARYNGECTOMIZED SPEAKERS ON SILENT BREATHING VERSUS SPEECH WITH ABDOMINAL AND CHEST AMPLITUDES IN MILLIMETERS

	Variables	$\bar{X}_{silence}$	$\bar{X}_{speech}$	$\bar{D}_{sil.-sp.}$	t
Normal N = 15	Abdominal amplitude	10.93	9.93	1.00	1.33
	Chest amplitude	12.42	13.11	-.69	.51
	Combined amplitude	11.68	11.52	.16	.20
Laryngec-tomized N = 15	Abdominal amplitude	13.32	9.49	3.83	2.58*
	Chest amplitude	17.12	11.33	5.79	4.26**
	Combined amplitude	15.25	10.41	4.84	4.28**

t df = 14
$t_{.01}$ = 2.977
$t_{.02}$ = 2.624
$t_{.05}$ = 2.145
** = .01
* = .05

significant. The difference between the abdominal amplitudes in silence and in speech with a t value of 2.58 is significant at the .02 level of confidence. The difference for the chest amplitudes in silence and in speech for the laryngectomized group with a t value of 4.26 is also significant at the .01 level of confidence.

Another important consideration concerns the possibility of differences between chest and abdominal amplitudes within each group as measured in silent breathing and as measured in speech breathing. Table 4 indicates that the normal group used greater chest amplitude than abdominal amplitude both in silence and in speech, but the difference of the chest and abdominal amplitudes is shown to be significant only for speech. The mean chest amplitude of 13.11 and the mean abdominal amplitude of 9.93 yields a difference of 3.18 and a t score of 2.19 which is significant at the .05 level of confidence.

The laryngectomized group also has greater chest amplitude than abdominal amplitude in silence and in speech, but the mean differences are not significant in either case.

Table 3 has indicated the mean amplitude difference $(\overline{D})$ between silence and speech within each group. The question arises as to whether or not the abdominal amplitude mean difference of 1.00 millimeter for the normal group differs significantly from the abdominal amplitude

TABLE 4

MEANS, MEAN DIFFERENCE, AND t VALUES WITHIN THE NORMAL AND LARYNGECTOMIZED SPEAKERS ON CHEST VERSUS ABDOMINAL IN SILENCE AND IN SPEECH, AMPLITUDE IN MILLIMETERS

	Variables	$\overline{X}_{chest}$	$\overline{X}_{abdom.}$	$\overline{D}_{ch.-ab.}$	t
Normal N = 15	Silence	12.42	10.93	1.49	1.28
	Speech	13.11	9.93	3.18	2.19*
Laryngec- tomized N = 15	Silence	17.12	13.32	3.80	1.98
	Speech	11.33	9.49	1.84	1.22

$$t\ df = 14$$
$$t_{.01} = 2.977$$
$$t_{.02} = 2.624$$
$$t_{.05} = 2.145$$
$$** = .01$$
$$* = .05$$

TABLE 5

DIFFERENCES BETWEEN NORMAL AND LARYNGECTOMIZED MEAN DIFFER-
ENCES OF SILENCE AND SPEECH BREATHING AMPLITUDES IN
MILLIMETERS FOR ABDOMINAL, CHEST, AND COMBINED
WITH MEANS AND t AND F VALUES

Normal N = 15 Laryngectomized N = 15	Abdominal		Chest		Combined	
	Norm.	Lar.	Norm.	Lar.	Norm.	Lar.
$\overline{X}_{speech}$	9.93	9.49	13.11	11.33	11.52	10.41
$\overline{X}_{silence}$	10.93	13.32	12.42	17.12	11.68	15.25
$\overline{D}_{sil. - sp.}$	1.00	3.83	- .69	5.79	.16	4.84
$\overline{D}_{lar.} - \overline{D}_{norm.}$	2.83		6.48		4.68	
t	1.70		3.41**		3.37**	
F	3.89**		1.04		2.03	

$$t \begin{cases} df = 28 \\ .01 = 2.763 \\ .02 = 2.467 \\ .05 = 2.048 \end{cases} \qquad F \begin{cases} df = 14 \text{ and } 14 \\ .02 = 3.70 \\ .05 = 3.34 \\ \text{(Interpolated)} \\ .10 = 2.48 \end{cases}$$

** = .01   ** = .02
* = .05   * = .05

mean difference of 3.83 for the laryngectomized group. Table 5 re-
arranges the D's for the convenience of showing the differences between
the mean differences and the resulting t and F scores. The abdominal
difference between the mean differences is not significant with a $\overline{D}$ of
2.83 and a t of 1.70. In chest amplitude and in combined amplitude
the differences between the normal and the laryngectomized mean differences in silence and in speech are significant. The difference of the
differences in chest amplitude, 6.48, gives a t value of 3.41, indicating
significance beyond the .01 level. Approximately the same situation
holds true for the combined amplitudes. Here the difference between

silence and speech for the normal group is .16 and for the laryngectomized group the difference is 4.84. The difference of the difference of 4.68 and the t value of 3.37 becomes significant beyond the .01 level of confidence. For the abdominal amplitude the difference between silence and speech for the normal group is 1.00 millimeter, while the difference for the laryngectomized group is 3.83. The difference of the differences, 2.83, in this case is not significant.

Table 6 indicates the difference between the differences for the abdominal and chest amplitudes in silence and speech for the two groups. The normal and the laryngectomized speakers do not differ significantly when comparison is made between the difference of the differences of the abdominal and chest amplitudes during silence and speech.

TABLE 6

DIFFERENCES BETWEEN NORMAL AND LARYNGECTOMIZED MEAN DIFFERENCES OF ABDOMINAL AND CHEST AMPLITUDES IN MILLIMETERS FOR SILENCE AND SPEECH WITH MEANS, t AND F VALUES

Normal N = 15 Laryngectomized N = 15	Silence		Speech	
	Norm.	Lar.	Norm.	Lar.
$\bar{X}_{abdominal}$	10.93	13.32	9.93	9.49
$\bar{X}_{chest}$	12.42	17.12	13.11	11.33
$\bar{D}_{chest-abdominal}$	1.49	3.80	3.18	1.84
$\bar{D}_{lar.} - \bar{D}_{norm.}$	2.31		-1.34	
t	1.03		.64	
F	2.70		1.08	

$$t \quad df = 28$$
$$t_{.01} = 2.763$$
$$t_{.02} = 2.467$$
$$t_{.05} = 2.048$$

$$F \quad df = 14 \text{ and } 14$$
$$F_{.02} = 3.70$$
$$F_{.05} = 3.34$$
$$\text{(Interpolated)}$$
$$F_{.10} = 2.48$$

THE FIVE-, SEVEN- AND NINE-SYLLABLE PHRASES

In order to obtain further samples of the speech coordinations employing different sentence lengths, phrases of five, seven and nine syllables were included in addition to the sixty-syllable paragraph for comparative purposes.

Figure 17 shows kymograms of the five-syllable phrase spoken by one laryngectomized and two normal speakers. Tracing I for the laryngectomized speaker S. L., judged to be highly intelligible, reveals a synchrony of movement between the movements of the chest (L. S.) and abdomen (Mes.), producing the five syllables in three phrases. The syllable pulses clearly show that the stress pattern is different for each syllable. The air pressure outside the mouth (A. O.) indicates that the speaker took two intakes of breath, as evidenced by the small, sharp dips in the line. The two normal speakers, A. L. in tracing II and W. P. in tracing III, spoke the five syllables in one phrase movement. The movements of the normals were smooth, regular and synchronous. The similarity of configuration is observable for the three speakers with the exception that speaker S. L. in tracing I spoke the five syllables in three phrases.

In Figure 18 the same three individuals speak a seven-syllable phrase. The two normal speakers produced the seven syllables in one phrase movement; but the laryngectomized speaker used three phrases to speak the seven syllables and took two intakes of air after he began speaking. Similarity between Figures 17 and 18 can be noted.

For Figure 19 the three speakers follow the same pattern as in Figure 17 and Figure 18, except that the laryngectomized speaker used four phrases in speaking the nine-syllable phrase.

Figures 20, 21 and 22 illustrate a laryngectomized speaker judged to be low in intelligibility speaking the five-, seven- and nine-syllable phrases respectively. The air pressure outside the mouth (A. O.) reveals an excessive number of intakes of air. The chest amplitude (L. S.) is exceptionally high in comparison to the abdominal amplitude. The five- and seven-syllable phrases are produced in three phrases and the nine syllables in four phrases. The phrasing movements are clearly differentiated in the chest movement and less differentiated in the abdominal movements. The chest and abdominal movements of this speaker appear to be out of phase. When a comparison is made between this speaker (Figures 20, 21 and 22), and the more intelligible laryngectomized speaker (S. L., I) in Figures 17, 18 and 19, differences in time in speaking the phrases are apparent. The poorer speaker used

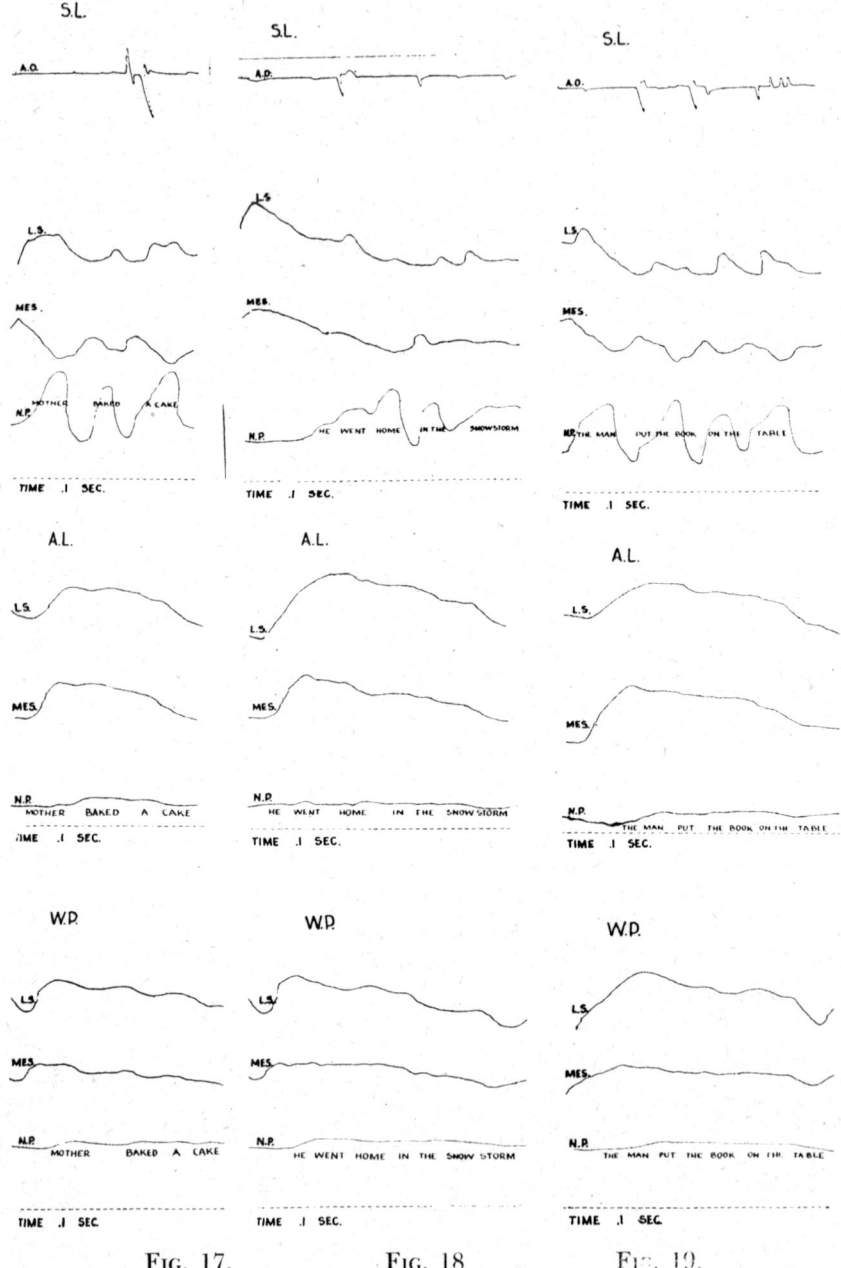

FIG. 17.   FIG. 18   FIG. 19.

FIG. 17. Kymograms of the five-syllable phrase spoken by one laryngectomized and two normal speakers.

I. *Subject:* S.L.—Laryngectomized speaker (High intelligibility).
  A.O. Tracing of the air pressure outside the mouth. The speaker takes two intakes of breath, as evidenced by the small sharp dips.
  L.S. Tracing of the movement of the chest wall, taken at the lower sternum. The tracing indicates that three phrases were used in speaking five syllables. Note the excessive amplitude for the first phrase, indicating an excessive amount of breath was employed.
  Mes. Tracing of the movement of the abdominal wall at the mesogastric level. The movements of the body walls appear to be synchronous.
  N.P. Tracing of the syllable pulse taken at the epigastric level. The stress for each syllable is different, indicating approach to normal rhythm.
II. *Subject:* A.L.—Normal speaker.
  L.S. Tracing of the movement of the chest wall, taken at the lower sternum. The five syllables are spoken on one smooth regular phrase.
  Mes. Tracing of the movement of the abdominal wall at the mesogastric level. Here as in the L.S., the five syllables are spoken on one smooth regular phrase.
  N.P. Tracing of the syllable pulse taken at the epigastric level. The syllables have definite stress, indicating normal patterns.
III. *Subject:* W.P.—Normal speaker.
  L.S. Tracing of the movement of the chest wall, taken at the lower sternum. The single phrase is smooth and regular.
  Mes. Tracing of the movement of the abdominal wall at the mesogastric level. The movement is smooth and regular in the tracings.
  N.P. Tracing of the syllable pulse taken at the epigastric level. The syllable stress indicates normal patterns.
        The essential difference between the laryngectomized speaker S.L., I, and the two normal speakers is that the five syllables were produced with a greater number of phrases.
Time is recorded in .1 seconds.

FIG. 18. Kymograms of the seven-syllable phrase spoken by one laryngectomized and two normal speakers.

I. *Subject:* S.L.—Laryngectomized speaker (High intelligibility).
  A.O. Tracing of the air pressure outside the mouth. The speaker takes two intakes of breath revealed by the two sharp dips in the line.
  L.S. Tracing of the movement of the chest wall, taken at the lower sternum. Three phrases were used in speaking the seven syllables. Note the similarity between this tracing and the speaker's production of the five-syllable phrase in Figure 17. There is greater chest pressure, however, in the tracing for the seven syllables.
  Mes. Tracing of the movement of the abdominal wall at the mesogastric level. The movement of the abdominal wall is synchronous with that of the chest, although there is less pressure evidenced.
  N.P. Tracing of the syllable pulse taken at the epigastric level. The stress for each syllable is different, indicating approach to normal rhythm.
II. *Subject:* A.L.—Normal speaker.
  L.S. Tracing of the movement of the chest wall, taken at the lower sternum. The seven syllables are spoken on one smooth regular phrase.

Fig. 18.—*Continued*

Mes. Tracing of the movement of the abdominal wall at the mesogastric level. Here as in the L.S. the seven syllables are spoken on one smooth regular phrase.

N.P. Tracing of the syllable pulse taken at the epigastric level. The syllables have definite stress patterns, indicating normal patterns.

Note the similarity between the speaker's production of the seven syllables and the five syllables in Figure 17.

III. *Subject:* W.P.—Normal speaker.

L.S. Tracing of the movement of the chest wall, taken at the lower sternum. The seven syllables are produced in one regular smooth phrase.

Mes. Tracing of the movement of the abdominal wall at the mesogastric level. The movement is smooth and regular in the tracing.

N.P. Tracing of the syllable pulse taken at the epigastric level. The syllable stress indicates normal patterns.

All three subjects took slightly longer to produce the seven syllables. But, the essential difference between the laryngectomized speaker, S.L., 1, and the two normal speakers is that the seven syllables were produced with a greater number of phrases by the laryngectomized speaker.

Time is recorded in .1 seconds.

Fig. 19. Kymograms of the nine-syllable phrase spoken by one laryngectomized and two normal speakers.

I. *Subject:* S.L.—Laryngectomized speaker (High intelligibility) .

A.O. Tracing of the air pressure outside the mouth. The speaker takes three distinct intakes of breath, as revealed by the sharp dips in the line.

L.S. Tracing of the movement of the chest wall taken at the lower sternum. The tracing indicates that four phrases were used in speaking nine syllables. Note the excessive amplitude for the first phrase, indicating an excessive amount of breath was employed.

Mes. Tracing of the movement of the abdominal wall at the mesogastric level. Note the synchronous behavior of the chest and abdominal walls.

N.P. Tracing of the syllable pulse taken at the epigastric level. The stress is different for each syllable, indicating approach to normal rhythm.

II. *Subject:* A.L.—Normal speaker.

L.S. Tracing of the movement of the chest wall, taken at the lower sternum. The nine syllables were spoken on one smooth regular phrase.

Mes. Tracing of the movement of the abdominal wall at the mesogastric level. Here as in the L.S., the nine syllables are spoken on one smooth regular phrase.

This speaker's productions of the five-, seven- and nine-syllable phrases are highly similar in configuration.

N.P. Tracing of the syllable pulse taken at the epigastric level. The syllables have definite stress patterns, indicating normal patterns.

III. *Subject:* W.P.—Normal speaker.

L.S. Tracing of the movement of the chest wall, taken at the lower sternum. The single phrase for the nine syllables is smooth and regular.

Mes. Tracing of the movement of the abdominal wall at the mesogastric level. The abdominal amplitude is not as great as the chest amplitude, which is characteristic for this speaker for the five, seven and nine syllables.

N.P. Tracing of the syllable pulse taken at the epigastric level. The syllable stress indicates normal patterns.

Fig. 19.—*Continued*

> The essential difference between the laryngectomized speaker S.L., I, and the two normal speakers is that the nine syllables were produced with a greater number of phrases.

Time is recorded in .1 seconds.

a considerably greater amount of time. His breathing movements are also less synchronous than the better laryngectomized speaker, and the better speaker more closely approximates the configurations of the normal speakers' tracings.

Table 7 summarizes the data for the five-syllable phrases. All of the normal subjects produced the five syllables in one phrase, while the laryngectomized individuals have a mean of 2.73 in number of phrases used to speak the five syllables. The difference between the two groups is significant beyond the .01 level of confidence.

In time taken to speak the phrase, the mean for the normal group is 2.41 seconds and for the laryngectomized group 3.08. The difference in this instance is significant at the .05 level of confidence. The differences between the variances of the two groups are also significant at the .02 level of confidence, with the laryngectomized group having a much larger variance.

A significant difference is found in the chest amplitude, with the normal group mean of 14.73 millimeters surpassing the laryngectomized mean of 8.94 millimeters. This difference is significant beyond the .01 level of confidence. In the combined amplitude approximately the same difference exists.

The results of the study of the seven-syllable phrases are found in Table 8. The mean time of 4.33 seconds taken by the laryngectomized group is significantly greater than the mean time for the normal group of 2.41 seconds beyond the .01 level of confidence. The seven syllables are still produced by the normal group in one phrase. The laryngectomized group used an average of 3.47 phrases. The difference continues to be significant beyond the .01 level of confidence.

There are no significant differences between the chest amplitudes and the abdominal amplitudes of the two groups.

The data for the nine-syllable phrases are found in Table 9. The mean of the time variable, 3.03 seconds for the normals and 5.13 seconds for the laryngectomized, yields a difference of 2.10 seconds and a t of 2.75, significant at the .05 level of confidence. The difference in number of phrases used to speak the nine syllables remains significant at the .01 level of confidence with the normal group maintaining the single phrase in speaking the nine syllables and the laryngectomized group offering a mean of 4.20 phrases.

J.K.

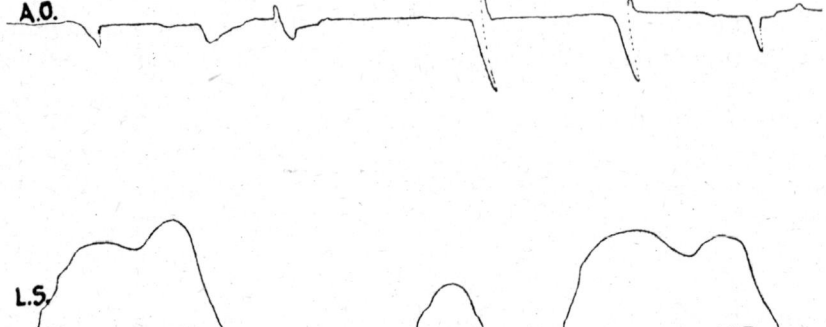

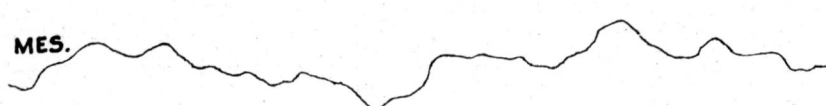

TIME .1 SEC.

FIG. 20. Kymogram of the five-syllable phrase spoken by a laryngectomized speaker.

I. *Subject:* J.K.—Laryngectomized speaker (Low intelligibility).

    A.O.   Tracing of the air pressure outside the mouth. Note the excessive number of intakes of air. There are six intakes of air revealed by the distinct dips in the line.

    L.S.   Tracing of the movement of the chest wall taken at the lower sternum.

Fig. 20.—*Continued*

The chest movement reveals three intakes of air in contrast to the six intakes pictured in the A.O. line. The chest pressure is excessive.

Mes. Tracing of the movement of the abdominal wall at the mesogastric level. The lower amplitude of the abdominal movement is contrasted with the L.S. line. The movements are out of phase with the chest movements, and a greater number of movements are noted in the abdominal line, substantiating the A.O. line.

N.P. No recording made.

Time is recorded in .1 seconds.

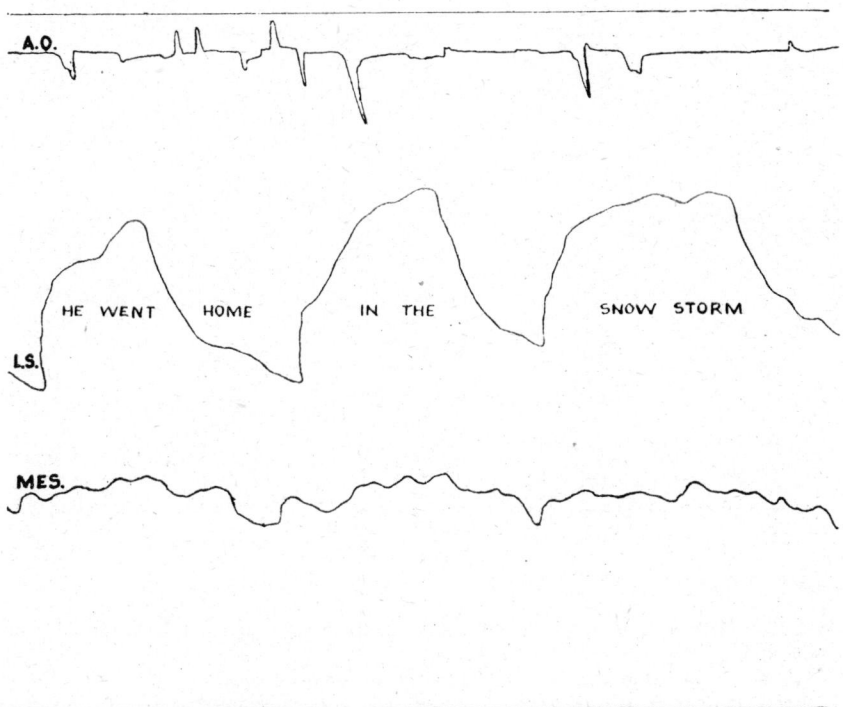

J.K.

A.O.

HE WENT   HOME   IN   THE   SNOW STORM

L.S.

MES.

TIME .1 SEC.

Fig. 21. Kymogram of the seven-syllable phrase spoken by a laryngectomized speaker.

I. *Subject:* J.K.—Laryngectomized speaker (Low intelligibility).

A.O. Tracing of the air pressure outside the mouth. Note the greater number of intakes in the A.O. line than in the L.S. line. There are six intakes of air.

L.S. Tracing of the movement of the chest wall taken at the lower sternum. The chest pressure is excessively high. There are three intakes of air in contrast to the six in the A.O. line.

Fig. 21.—*Continued*

Mes. Tracing of the movement of the abdominal wall at the mesogastric level.
The smaller amplitude of the abdominal movement is contrasted with the
L.S. line. The movements are out of phase with the chest movements, and
a greater number of movements are noted in the abdominal line, substantiating the A.O. line.

N.P. No recording made.

Time is recorded in .1 seconds.

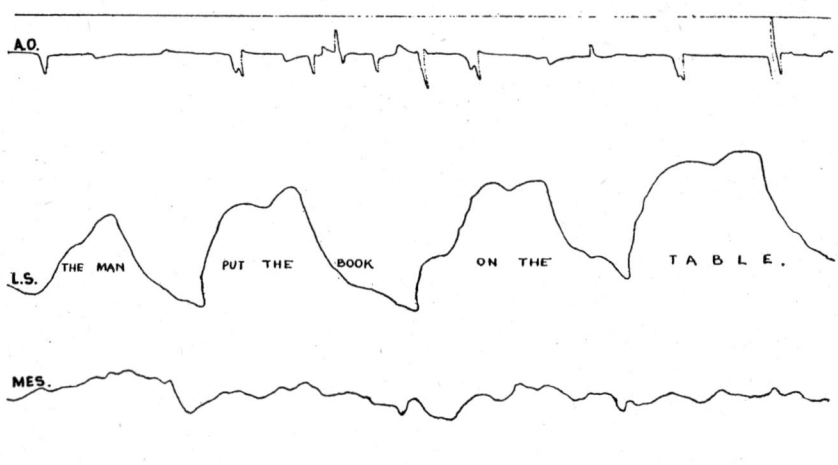

Fig. 22. Kymogram of the nine-syllable phrase spoken by a laryngectomized
speaker.

I. *Subject:* J.K.—Laryngectomized speaker (Low intelligibility).

A.O. Tracing of the air pressure outside the mouth. Note the excessive number
of intakes of air. The tracing reveals eleven intakes of air.

L.S. Tracing of the movement of the chest wall taken at the lower sternum.
The chest movement reveals four intakes of air, while the A.O. line indicates
eleven intakes of air, three of these between phrases two and three, indicating
that he is taking in air without accompanying speech. Great amplitude for
the chest indicates an excessive amount of breath is being used.

Mes. Tracing of the movement of the abdominal wall at the mesogastric level.
The great difference in amplitude between the abdominal and chest amplitude is indicated. The greater number of movements of the abdominal line
are out of phase with the chest movements. This line more closely approximates the A.O. line than the chest line (L.S.).

N.P. No recording made.

Time is recorded in .1 seconds.

TABLE 7

MEANS, VARIANCES, STANDARD DEVIATIONS, DIFFERENCES BETWEEN THE MEANS, t
AND F VALUES FOR SPEECH BREATHING OF THE NORMAL AND LARYNGECTOMIZED
SPEAKERS ON THE FIVE-SYLLABLE PHRASES FOR TIME, NUMBER OF
PHRASES, TIME PER PHRASE, NUMBER OF SYLLABLES, AND
FOR ABDOMINAL, CHEST AND COMBINED AMPLITUDES
IN MILLIMETERS

Variables	Normal			Laryngectomized			$\bar{X}_{lar.}-\bar{X}_{n.}$	t	F
	$\bar{X}$	σ^2	σ	$\bar{X}$	σ^2	σ			
Time	2.41	.21	.46	3.08	1.09	1.04	.67	2.28^x	5.18**
No. of phrases	1.00			2.73	1.50	1.22	1.73	5.48**	
Time per phrase				1.29	.25	.50			
No. of syllables	5.00			2.37	2.06	1.44			
Abdominal amplitude	10.77	36.25	6.02	7.67	8.86	2.98	-3.10	1.79	4.09**
Chest amplitude	14.73	32.50	5.70	8.94	15.60	3.95	-5.79	3.23**	2.08
Combined amplitude	12.75	22.97	4.79	8.31	9.67	3.11	-4.44	3.01**	2.38

n. = Normal speakers
lar. = Laryngectomized speakers

x = .05 Indicates signif-
  icance of t when
  F is significant

df = 28
$t_{.01}$ = 2.763
$t_{.02}$ = 2.467
$t_{.05}$ = 2.048
df = 14
$t_{.01}$ = 2.977
$t_{.02}$ = 2.624
$t_{.05}$ = 2.145

** = .01
* = .05

df = 14 and 14
$F_{.02}$ = 3.70
$F_{.05}$ = 3.34
(Interpolated)
$F_{.10}$ = 2.48

** = .02
* = .05

In mean abdominal amplitude a significant difference at the .01 level of confidence appears between the normal and the laryngectomized groups, with the normals having the greater mean amplitude of 13.07 millimeters and the laryngectomized group a mean of 7.44 millimeters. The chest amplitude for the normals of 15.87 millimeters is significantly greater at the .01 level of confidence than the 10.33 mean of the laryngectomized individuals. As might be expected, the combined amplitudes of the two groups are also significantly different.

The results of the study of the five-, seven- and nine-syllable phrases can readily be compared to the results of the sixty-syllable paragraph. It was found that time and number of phrases differentiate the two

TABLE 8

MEANS, VARIANCES, STANDARD DEVIATIONS, DIFFERENCES BETWEEN THE MEANS, t
AND F VALUES FOR SPEECH BREATHING OF THE NORMAL AND LARYNGECTOMIZED
SPEAKERS ON THE SEVEN-SYLLABLE PHRASES FOR TIME, NUMBER OF
PHRASES, TIME PER PHRASE, NUMBER OF SYLLABLES, AND
FOR ABDOMINAL, CHEST AND COMBINED AMPLITUDES
IN MILLIMETERS

Variables	Normal			Laryngectomized			$\overline{X}_{lar.}\overline{X}_{n.}$	t	F
	$\overline{X}$	σ^2	σ	$\overline{X}$	σ^2	σ			
Time	2.77	.22	.47	4.33	3.44	1.85	.67	3.16^{xx}	15.57^{**}
No. of phrases	1.00			3.47	2.56	1.60	2.47	5.99^{**}	
Time per phrase				1.42	.32	.56			
No. of syllables	7.00			2.75	3.64	1.91			
Abdominal amplitude	11.33	32.67	5.72	8.40	14.81	3.85	-2.93	1.65	2.21
Chest amplitude	15.60	26.94	5.19	11.41	42.01	6.48	-4.19	1.95	1.56
Combined amplitude	13.54	18.55	4.31	9.91	18.77	4.33	-4.44	2.30^{*}	1.01

```
      n. = Normal speakers                df = 28            df = 14 and 14
    lar. = Laryngectomized speakers     t.01 = 2.763    F.02 = 3.70
                                         t.02 = 2.467    F.05 = 3.34
      xx = .01 Indicates signif-        t.05 = 2.048    (Interpolated)
       x = .05 icance of t when           df = 14        F.10 = 2.48
               F  is significant        t.01 = 2.977
                                         t.02 = 2.624    ** = .02
                                         t.05 = 2.145     * = .05

                                         ** = .01
                                          * = .05
```

groups significantly. In each case the laryngectomized individuals used
greater time and employed a greater number of phrases in speaking.

In the sixty-syllable paragraph none of the amplitude measurements
reveal any significant difference between the two groups. But, the mean
values for the normal group are higher in abdominal, chest and combined amplitudes. This same trend is revealed in the five-, seven- and
nine-syllable phrases. Significant differences are shown, however, in:

1. abdominal amplitude in the nine-syllable phrase,
2. chest amplitude in the five- and nine-syllable phrase,
3. and in the combined amplitudes for the three phrases.

The normal speakers all produced the five-, seven- and nine-syllable
phrases on one phrasing movement. But, the mean number of phrases

TABLE 9

MEANS, VARIANCES, STANDARD DEVIATIONS, DIFFERENCES BETWEEN THE MEANS, t AND F VALUES FOR SPEECH BREATHING OF THE NORMAL AND LARYNGECTOMIZED SPEAKERS ON THE NINE-SYLLABLE PHRASES FOR TIME, NUMBER OF PHRASES, TIME PER PHRASE, NUMBER OF SYLLABLES, AND FOR ABDOMINAL, CHEST AND COMBINED AMPLITUDES IN MILLIMETERS

Variables	Normal			Laryngectomized			$\bar{X}_{lar.}-\bar{X}_{n.}$	t	F
	$\bar{X}$	σ^2	σ	$\bar{X}$	σ^2	σ			
Time	3.03	.21	.45	5.13	8.56	2.93	2.10	2.75ˣ	41.74**
No. of phrases	1.00			4.20	5.17	2.27	5.45	5.45**	
Time per phrase				1.38	.38	.62			
No. of syllables	9.00			3.15	6.41	2.53			
Abdominal amplitude	13.07	38.32	6.19	7.44	13.10	3.62	-5.63	3.04**	2.92
Chest amplitude	15.87	24.27	4.93	10.33	20.29	4.50	-5.54	3.21**	1.20
Combined amplitude	14.47	17.17	4.14	8.88	10.49	3.24	-5.59	4.12**	1.64

n. = Normal speakers
lar. = Laryngectomized speakers

xx = .01 Indicates signif-
x = .05 icance of t when
F is significant

df = 28
$t_{.01}$ = 2.763
$t_{.02}$ = 2.467
$t_{.05}$ = 2.048
df = 14
$t_{.01}$ = 2.977
$t_{.02}$ = 2.624
$t_{.05}$ = 2.145

** = .01
* = .05

df = 14 and 14
$F_{.02}$ = 3.70
$F_{.05}$ = 3.34
(Interpolated)
$F_{.10}$ = 2.48

** = .02
* = .05

employed by the laryngectomized speakers for the five-, seven- and nine-syllable phrases were 2.73, 3.47 and 4.20 phrases respectively.

The speech coordinations of the normal and laryngectomized speakers have been examined in the light of Stetson's hypothesis that there is no difference between the two groups. Stetson's (57) laryngectomized speakers were employing excellent "oesophageal speech." The statistical analysis in the present study has revealed some differences to exist between the two groups. The inspection of the individual kymograms, however, reveals similarities in the configuration patterns between the laryngectomized speakers judged to be high in intelligibility and the normal speakers.

Statistical analysis of the speech coordination data for the normal and the laryngectomized speakers reveals the following significant differences.

The laryngectomized speakers as a group:

1. employed more time in speaking the speech samples,
2. employed a greater number of phrases in speaking.

The kymograms shown in Figures 23 through 27 illustrate further the similarities and differences found in the speech coordinations of the two groups. In Figure 23 the air pressure outside the mouth as well as the tracings of the lower sternum area and of the mesogastric area, including the syllable pulse, are shown for one normal and one laryngectomized speaker. The air pressure outside the mouth (A. O.) for the normal subject (W. W., in tracing I) shows three dips in the line indicating the intake of air, corresponding to the three beginning phrasing movements at the lower sternum area and at the mesogastric level. For the laryngectomized subject, (S. L., in tracing II) the A. O. line reveals a great many more intakes of breath, corresponding to the beginning phrase movements in the lower sternum and the mesogastric regions. The phrasing movements are synchronous.

Figure 24 reveals the air pressure tracings taken just outside the mouth during the speaking of the groups of syllables by two normal speakers and two laryngectomized speakers. The normal speakers, A. P., in tracing I, and D. C., in tracing II, reveal characteristic outside-the-mouth air pressures, showing the absence of the aspiration phase for the first four syllables [ɑ] [ɑ] [ɑ] [ɑ], and a clear aspiration phase in the second and third group of syllables, indicating the function of the releasing consonant [h]. The two laryngectomized speakers, S. L., in tracing III, and P. S., in tracing IV, show the releasing consonant function in the first group of syllables [ɑ] [ɑ] [ɑ] [ɑ]. The downward excursions in the line indicate the intake of breath on the part of the laryngectomized individuals before each syllable. The normals do not reveal these downward excursions or the releasing consonant functions.

For the second and third groups of syllables the [hɑ] [hɑ] [hɑ] [hɑ] and [hɑ-ɑ] [hɑ-ɑ] [hɑ-ɑ] [hɑ-ɑ] there is a greater extent of intake as indicated by the downward excursion on the part of the laryngectomized speakers. There is little difference shown in the speaking of the [hɑ] and the [hɑ-ɑ] groups indicating voicing throughout.

Figures 25 and 26 reveal the air pressure inside the mouth during the articulation of groups of syllables consisting of releasing and arresting consonants for the two normal and two laryngectomized speakers. In Figure 25 the normal speakers, G. H., in tracing I, and A. P., in tracing II, illustrate the differential pressure rises for the [bʌ] and [ʌb] as compared with the [pʌ] and [ʌp]. The pressure for the [pʌ] and [ʌp] group

I W.W.

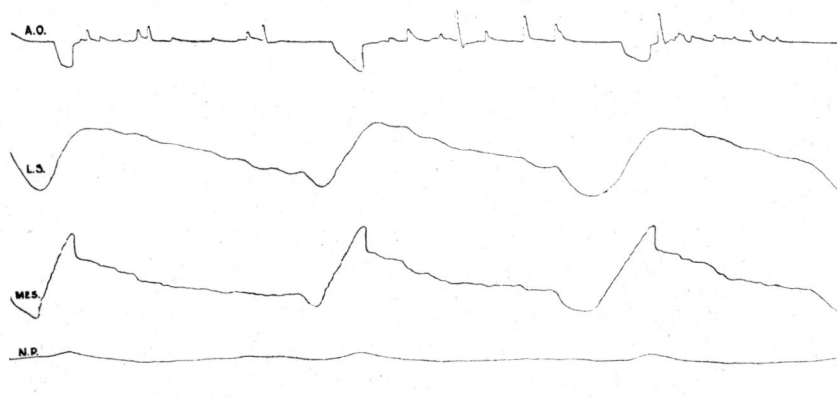

II S.L.

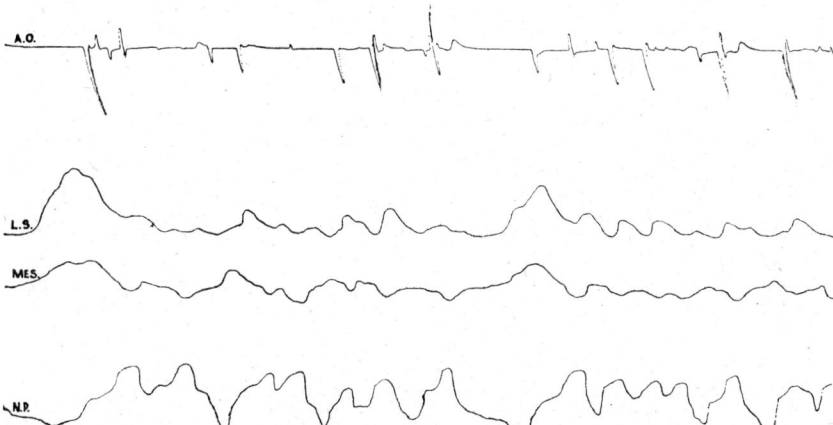

FIG. 23. Kymograms of the sixty-syllable paragraph spoken by one normal speaker and one laryngectomized speaker, showing tracings of the air pressure outside of the mouth, the movement of the chest wall taken at the lower sternum, the movement of the abdominal wall taken at the mesogastric area, and the tracing of the syllable pulse.

I. *Subject:* W.W.—Normal speaker.

A.O. Tracing of the air pressure outside the mouth. Note the dips indicating the intake of air at the beginning of each phrase. The upward movements of the tracings indicate vowels spoken. There are three intakes of air corresponding to the three beginning phrasing movements indicated in the L.S. and the Mes. lines.

Fig. 23.—*Continued*

L.S.   Tracing of the movement of the chest wall, taken at the lower sternum. Three normal phrasing movements are indicated, which are synchronous with the three intakes of air in the A.O. line.

Mes.   Tracing of the movement of the abdominal wall at the mesogastric level. Three normal phrasing movements in synchrony with the chest and outside the mouth pressure lines are indicated.

N.P.   Tracing of the syllable pulse taken at the epigastric level. The distinct syllable pulses are indicated.

II. *Subject:* S.L.—Laryngectomized speaker (High intelligibility).

A.O.   Tracing of the air pressure outside the mouth. Downward movements indicate intakes of breath which correspond to the beginning phrase movements in the L.S. and Mes. tracings.

L.S.   Tracing of the movement of the chest wall, taken at the lower sternum. Note the greater number of phrases and irregularity of movement with the large amplitudes at certain phrases indicating large expenditure of breath.

Mes.   Tracing of the movement of the abdominal wall at the mesogastric level. Note the greater number of phrases which coincide with chest movements in the L.S. line.

N.P.   Tracing of the syllable pulse taken at the epigastric level. Note the irregularity of the stress for each syllable indicating division of syllables into feet.

Time is recorded in .1 seconds.

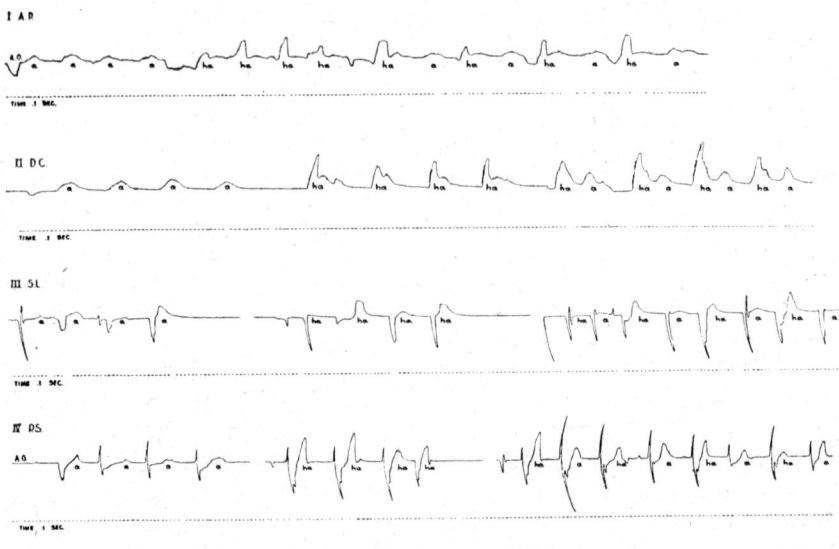

Fig. 24. Kymograms of the air pressure tracings just outside the mouth during groups of syllables for two normal and two laryngectomized speakers.

   Syllables: [ɑ] [ɑ] [ɑ] [ɑ];   [hɑ] [hɑ] [hɑ] [hɑ];
                  [hɑ-ɑ] [hɑ-ɑ] [hɑ-ɑ] [hɑ-ɑ]

'I. *Subject:* A.P.—Normal speaker.

A.O.   Tracing of the air pressure outside the mouth. Note the aspiration phase

Fig. 24.—*Continued*

is absent in the first four syllables [ɑ] [ɑ] [ɑ] [ɑ]. The rise in pressure of the syllables without returning to the base line between syllables indicates that the four syllables are spoken on a phrase. For the [hɑ] [hɑ] [hɑ] [hɑ], the aspiration phase increases indicating the function of the releasing consonant of the [h]. In speaking the [hɑ-ɑ] series, the aspiration phrase increases for the [h] and decreases for the [ɑ], indicating that the [h] in the [hɑ] functions as a releasing consonant.

II. *Subject:* D.C.—Normal speaker.

A.O.   Tracing of the air pressure outside the mouth. Note the aspiration phase is absent in the first four syllables, [ɑ] [ɑ] [ɑ] [ɑ]. The rise in pressure of the syllables without returning to the base line between syllables indicates that the four syllables are spoken on a phrase. For the [hɑ] series, the aspiration phase increases indicating the function of the releasing consonant of the [h]. In speaking the [hɑ-ɑ] series, the aspiration phase increases for the [hɑ] and decreases for the [ɑ], indicating that the [hɑ] in the [hɑ-ɑ] functions as a releasing consonant.

III. *Subject:* S.L.—Laryngectomized speaker (High intelligibility).

A.O.   Tracing of the air pressure outside the mouth. Note the intakes of air by the downward excursion before each syllable. In the first group, the [ɑ] series, the final [ɑ] is spoken with great pressure. For the [hɑ] series the speaker inhales before each syllable. The tracings for the first and third syllables reveal no consonantal function, while the second and fourth syllables indicate a consonantal function. The tracings for the [hɑ-ɑ] series also reveal an intake of air by downward excursion of the tracing before each syllable. The tracings are pronounced and show greater intake than for the [ɑ] group. The consonantal function appears reduced in this group indicating probable voicing throughout.

IV. *Subject:* P.S.—Laryngectomized speaker (High intelligibility).

A.O.   Tracing of the air pressure outside the mouth. Note the intakes of air by the downward excursion before each syllable. In the first group, the [ɑ] series, the final [ɑ] is spoken with great pressure. For the [hɑ] group the releasing consonant function is clear for the four syllables. All the four syllables were voiced by the speaker. For the [hɑ-ɑ] group again the downward excursions of the tracing reveal intakes of air. There is little difference between the [hɑ] and the [ɑ], indicating voicing throughout.

is much greater than for the [bʌ] and [ʌb] groups. The laryngectomized speakers, O. R., in tracing III, and H. G., in tracing IV, do not show the characteristic differential in pressures as do the normal speakers. There is very little pressure difference between any of the groups which indicates that the speakers do not differentiate between the surd and the sonant group.

Figure 26, like 25, illustrates kymograms of the air pressure inside the mouth taken while the subject is speaking groups of four syllables. For the normal subjects the air pressure inside the mouth is very little for the [ɑ] series since the mouth is open when these syllables are being spoken. For the [hɑ] there is an aspiration phase increase reflecting the operational efficiency of the releasing consonant. The [hɑ-ɑ] groups reveal an aspiration phase for the releasing consonant and a dropping of the pressure for the [ɑ]. For the laryngectomized subjects, P. S., in tracing III, and S. L., in tracing IV, the excessively high pressures are noted for the syllable groupings. There is no differentiation for the change of the air pressure in the mouth. The vocalization of the [ɑ] is preceded by

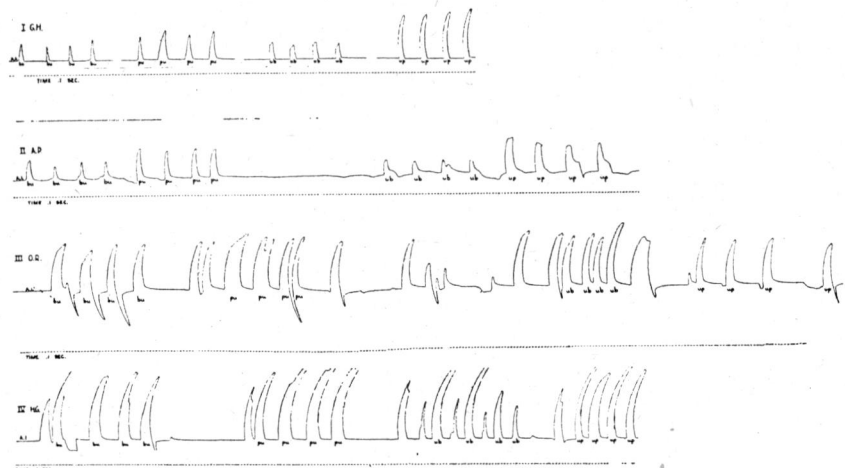

Fɪɢ. 25. Kymograms of the air pressure inside the mouth during articulation of groups of syllables consisting of releasing and arresting consonants for two normal and two laryngectomized speakers.

*Vowel sound in above tracing is [ʌ] rather than [ʊ].

Syllables: [bʌ] [bʌ] [bʌ] [bʌ]; [pʌ] [pʌ] [pʌ] [pʌ];
             [ʌb] [ʌb] [ʌb] [ʌb]; [ʌp] [ʌp] [ʌp] [ʌp].

I. Subject: G.H.—Normal speaker.
  A.I.   Tracing of the air pressure inside the mouth. The differential in air pressures for the [bʌ] and [pʌ] is clearly indicated. The greater pressure for the surd is indicated. This situation holds for the [ʌb] and the [ʌp] as well.

II. Subject: A.P.—Normal speaker.
  A.I.   Tracing of the air pressure inside the mouth. The differential in air pressures for the [bʌ] and [pʌ] is clearly indicated, the greater pressure for the surd. This situation holds for the [ʌb] and the [ʌp] as well.

III. Subject: O.R.—Laryngectomized speaker (Low intelligibility).
  A.I.   Tracing of the air pressure inside the mouth. The characteristic differential pressures betwen the sonant and the surd is not revealed. There is no differentiation throughout the entire series. Those tracings not marked are the speaker's attempts to inhale air, which do not fuse with the beginning of the syllable. Note the negative pressures.

IV. Subject: H.G.—Laryngectomized speaker (High intelligibility).
  A.I.   Tracing of the air pressure inside the mouth. The characteristic differential pressures between the sonant and the surd is not revealed. There is no differentiation throughout the cntire series. Those tracings not marked are the speaker's attempts to inhale air, which do not fuse with the beginning of the syllable. Note also the lack of differentiation between the [ʌb] and the [ʌp] groups.

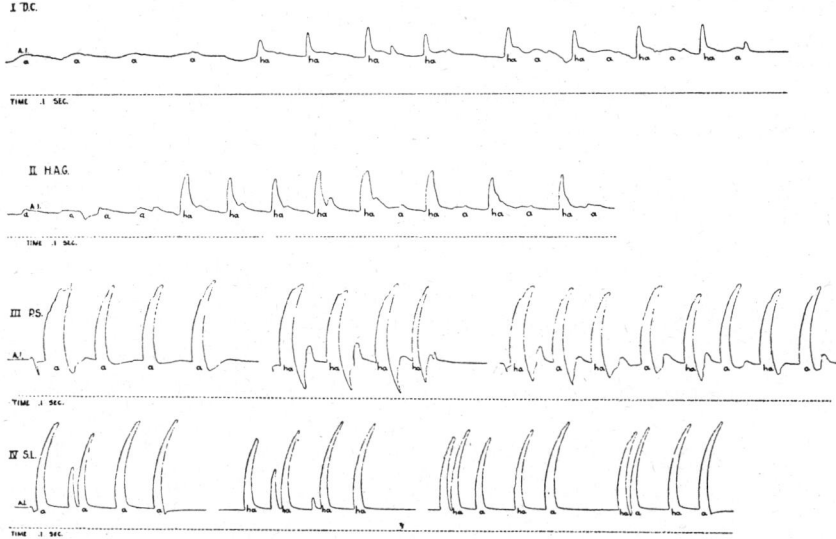

Fig. 26. Kymograms of the air pressure inside the mouth during three groups of syllables consisting of one group possessing neither releasing nor arresting consonants, a second group containing a releasing consonant and a third series of two syllable groupings, the first syllable containing a releasing consonant and the second containing neither a releasing nor an arresting consonant.

    Syllables: [ɑ] [ɑ] [ɑ] [ɑ]; [hɑ] [hɑ] [hɑ] [hɑ];
                [hɑ-ɑ] [hɑ-ɑ] [hɑ-ɑ] [hɑ-ɑ].

I. *Subject:* D.C.—Normal speaker.
    A.I.   Tracing of the air pressure inside the mouth. There is very little pressure for the [ɑ] group, since the mouth is open when these syllables are being produced. For the [hɑ] group the aspiration phase indicates reflecting the operational efficiency of the releasing consonant. The [hɑ-ɑ] group reveals an aspiration phase for the releasing consonant and a dropping of pressure for the [ɑ].

II. *Subject:* H.A.G.—Normal speaker.
    A.I.   Tracing of the air pressure inside the mouth. There is very little pressure for the group, since the mouth is open when these syllables are being produced. For the [hɑ] group the aspiration phase increases reflecting the operational efficiency of the releasing consonant. The [hɑ-ɑ] group reveals an aspiration phase for the releasing consonant and a dropping of pressure for the [ɑ]. Note the slightly greater pressure for the [ɑ] group in contrast to the above speaker, D.C.

III. *Subject:* P.S.—Laryngectomized speaker (High intelligibility).
    A.I.   Tracing of the air pressure inside the mouth. Note the excessive pressure for the entire syllable group. There is no differentiation in terms of air pressure in the mouth. In the [ɑ] group the vocalization of the [ɑ] is preceded by releasing consonant, indicating that the speaker closes his mouth and builds pressure previous to releasing the [ɑ]. The tracing reveals that the vocalization is actually [bɑ]. In the [hɑ] group the [ɑ]'s

FIG. 26.–*Continued*

are preceded by high pressure in the mouth previous to the releasing of the [ɑ]. The laryngectomized speaker brings his lips together and builds up pressure previous to releasing the syllable. The syllable is actually [bɑ]. The [hɑ-ɑ] group reveals the same phenomena as the [hɑ] and the [ɑ] groups. There is a negative pressure between each syllable indicating that each syllable spoken as a phrase and that excessive amounts of pressure are used in speaking the syllable.

IV. *Subject:* S.L.–Laryngectomized speaker (High intelligibility).

A.I.   Tracing of the aid pressure inside the mouth. In the [ɑ] group the laryngectomized speaker closes his mouth to build pressure before releasing the syllable. Before the first and second [ɑ]'s there is a rising of pressure without vocalization. For the [hɑ] group the pressure is excessive revealing the closure of the lips previous to vocalizing the [ɑ]. Between the first and second and the second and third syllables there are two pressure rises unaccompanied by vocalization. For the [hɑ-ɑ] group there is a rise of pressure before the speaking of the syllables. The pressures for the [hɑ] and the [ɑ] are approximately the same indicating closure of the lips before vocalization. Note the similarity of tracings for all groups indicating that the speaker is actually saying [bɑ].

the releasing consonant indicating that the laryngectomized speaker closes his mouth and builds pressure previous to releasing the [ɑ]. The tracings reveal that the vocalization is [bɑ]. The same situation holds for the remaining two groups, [hɑ] and [hɑ-ɑ].

Stetson (51) in his research with laryngectomized individuals who had learned "oesophageal speech" indicated that the original chest movements for speech persist and that the chest pulses continue to be produced and that they are comparable to the syllable pulse obtained by the negative pressure apparatus. He tapped this pressure sub-glottally. Figure 27 indicates kymograms of the sub-glottal air pressure and the syllable pulse in groups of syllables for three laryngectomized speakers. A tracing of the air flow in the trachea was obtained by enclosing the tracheal stoma with an "embouchure." There is distinct movement for each syllable. The tracings for the three speakers indicate that the syllable pulses taken at the epigastric level are clearly shown and coincide with the tracings taken at the sub-glottal position, revealing that the chest pulse is continued and is measurable by the air pressures in the trachea.

INTELLIGIBILITY

A preliminary pilot investigation was undertaken to ascertain if significant differences would occur in the speech intelligibility scores of the laryngectomized persons if the speech materials were tape recorded under the following two conditions:

1. a kymograph-recording position (Figures 5 and 6),
2. a tape-recording position in a sound-treated room (Figure 7).

Tape recordings of speech materials (ten sentences) were made for four laryngectomized speakers in both conditions. These tape recordings were then judged for intelligibility by two groups of seven speech pathology and audiology majors. The mean intelligibility score for the four laryngectomized for position I (kymograph) is 76.13 per cent, for position II (sound-treated room) 76.74 per cent, the mean difference being −.61. The t value for the difference is .12. It is felt that no meaningful difference exists in relation to the scores obtained in the two positions. The number of subjects employed in the pilot study was small, however, Cypreansen (9) in the same type of pilot study with four cerebral palsied children found similar results.

The tape-recording position in the sound-treated room (Figure 7) was employed for recording of speech materials for the laryngectomized subjects.

It is hypothesized:

1. that the quantitative intelligibility indexes employed in this investigation would differentiate between the laryngectomized speakers;

2. that the most intelligible laryngectomized speakers would approximate more closely the speech coordinations of the normal speakers.

In making judgments of intelligibility, it becomes necessary to determine the type of auditors to be utilized. In the present study two different types of auditors were employed:

1. university students who were speech pathology and audiology majors,

2. students who were non-speech pathology and audiology majors.

It was desirable to discover if these two groups differed in judging the speech intelligibility of laryngectomized individuals. Table 10 shows the results of a comparison of the two auditing groups. It is revealed that the two groups differ significantly beyond the .01 level of confidence on all three intelligibility criteria, PB's, multiple choice and sentences. Although the speech pathology and audiology majors give higher mean scores for each criterion, the high correlations, above .96 in each case, reveal that either group of auditors differentiates the laryngectomized speakers in an almost identical manner on the basis of intelligibility. Since there appears to be no justification in combining the two groups of auditing scores, a decision was made to employ only the speech pathology and audiology majors' auditing scores. It was felt that these auditors because of their training in listening and sound discrimination would not unduly penalize the laryngectomized speakers.

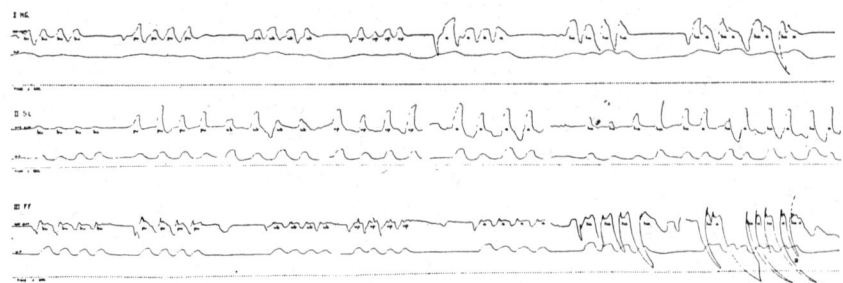

FIG. 27. Kymograms of the sub-glottal air pressure and the syllable pulse during groups of syllables for three laryngectomized speakers.

*Vowel sound in above tracing is [ʌ] rather than [ʊ].

I. *Subject:* H.G.—Laryngectomized speaker (High intelligibility).

Syllables: Groups [bʌ]; [pʌ]; [ʌb]; [ʌp]; [ɑ]; [hɑ]; [hɑ-ɑ].

Sub-glott. Tracing of the air flow in the trachea, obtained by the enclosing of the tracheal stoma in an embouchure. Note there is a distinct movement for each syllable. Also the pressure for the first four groups is even and regular. For the group [ɑ], [hɑ] and [hɑ-ɑ], the pressure is much greater indicating excessive amounts of escaping air from the tracheal stoma. In addition there is greater downward excursion for the [hɑ] and the [hɑ-ɑ] groups between syllables indicating intakes of air at the syllable junctures.

N.P. Tracing of the syllable pulse taken at the epigastric level. The individual syllables are clearly shown and coincide exactly with the movements as revealed by the sub-glottal tracings. The regularity of occurrence of this phenomena permits one to substitute sub-glottal pulses for the syllable pulses. The speaker breaks the [hɑ-ɑ] group into four groups. The syllable pulses show accent on the first [hɑ] and the last three [ɑ]'s. This would reveal an iambic pentameter pattern. The [hɑ-ɑ]'s are grouped into feet of two syllables each.

II. *Subject:* S.L.—Laryngectomized speaker (High intelligibility).

Sub-glott. Tracing of the air flow in the trachea, obtained by the enclosing of the tracheal stoma in an embouchure. Note the variations in air pressure for the speaker. Note that the individual syllables are clearly marked.

N.P. Tracing of the syllable pulse taken at the epigastric level. Note the regularity and the unequivocal syllable pulses revealed by the tracings.

III. *Subject:* F.F.—Laryngectomized speaker (Low intelligibility).

Sub-glott. Tracing of the air flow in the trachea, obtained by the enclosing of the tracheal stoma in an embouchure. The pressure pulses are approximately equal throughout all the groups, but the [hɑ] and the [hɑ-ɑ] group reveal distinct negative pressures, indicated by the downward dips in the line. The tracing reflects that each syllable is spoken as a phrase.

N.P. This tracing reveals clear and distinct syllable pulses. Each syllable receives practically the same stress. The speech tends to be monotonous.

TABLE 10

MEANS, VARIANCES, STANDARD DEVIATIONS, F, MEAN DIFFERENCES, AND
t, r, AND r^2 FOR SPEECH PATHOLOGY AND AUDIOLOGY MAJORS AND
NON-SPEECH PATHOLOGY AND AUDIOLOGY MAJORS AS AUDITORS OF
PB LISTS, MULTIPLE CHOICE TEST, AND SENTENCES
WITH SCORES IN PERCENT CORRECT

N = 15		$\overline{X}$	σ^2	σ	F	$\overline{D}$	t	r	r^2
PB Words	Speech Pathology	44.88	589.88	24.28	1.01	6.15	3.75**	.9658**	.9328
	Non-Speech Pathology	38.73	595.21	24.40					
Multiple Choice	Speech Pathology	75.53	237.55	15.41	1.08	4.07	4.51**	.9761**	.9528
	Non-Speech Pathology	71.47	257.12	16.00					
Sentences	Speech Pathology	67.63	1,002.89	31.67	1.01	9.25	4.11**	.9625**	.9264
	Non-Speech Pathology	58.38	1,017.92	31.90					

df = 14
$t_{.01}$ = 2.977
$t_{.02}$ = 2.624
$t_{.05}$ = 2.145
df = 13
$r_{.01}$ = .641
$r_{.05}$ = .514

** = .01

Figures 28, 29 and 30 are scatter diagrams and distributions indicating the relationship between speech pathology and audiology majors and non-speech pathology and audiology majors as auditors in judging the intelligibility of laryngectomized individuals. The three criteria are PB's, multiple choice intelligibility test and sentences. The high linear relationships are readily observable between the two auditing groups. The frequency distributions, although illustrating higher means for the speech pathology and audiology majors, also reveal marked similarity in the variability of the groups. The two groups of auditors are highly comparable in their ability to differentiate the laryngectomized speakers on the basis of intelligibility.

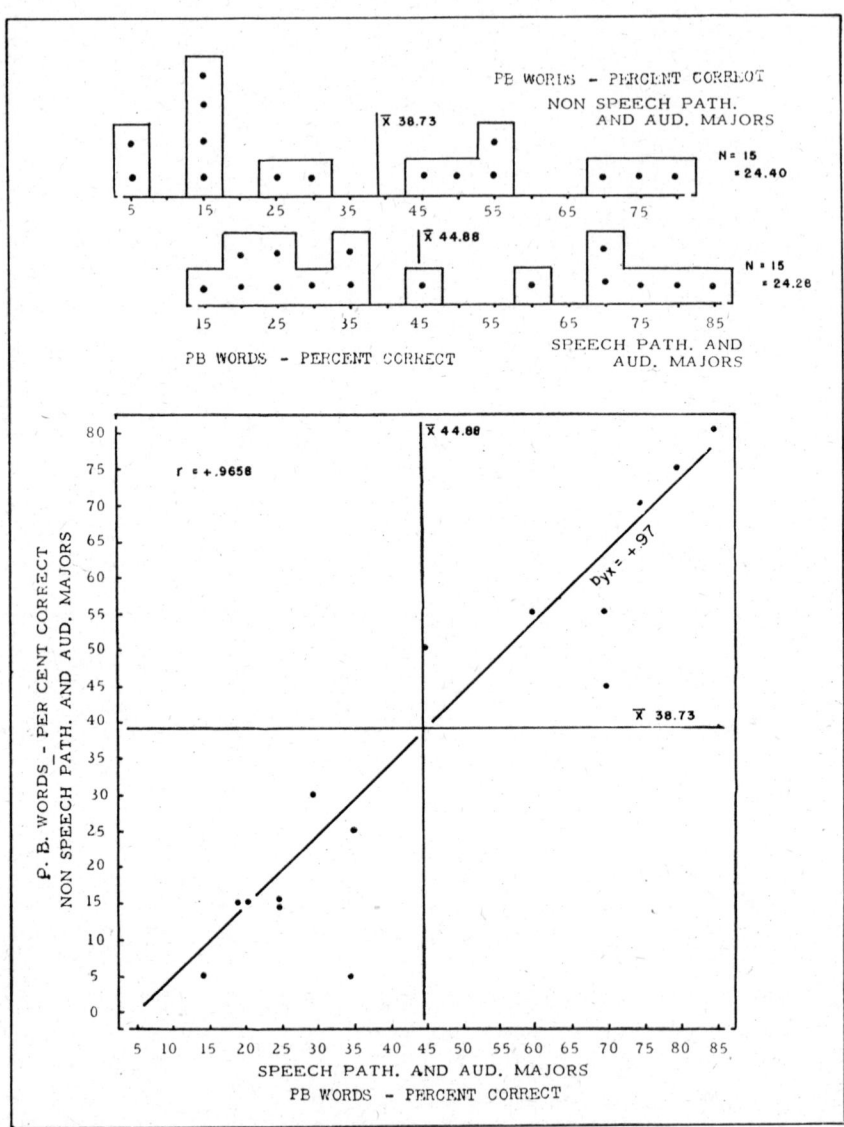

FIG. 28. Scatter diagram showing auditing scores of the speech pathology and audiology and the non-speech pathology and audiology majors on the PB words in per cent correct in relation to the laryngectomized group, giving means, regression line, and Pearson r, and also showing distribution of scores for the two auditing groups.

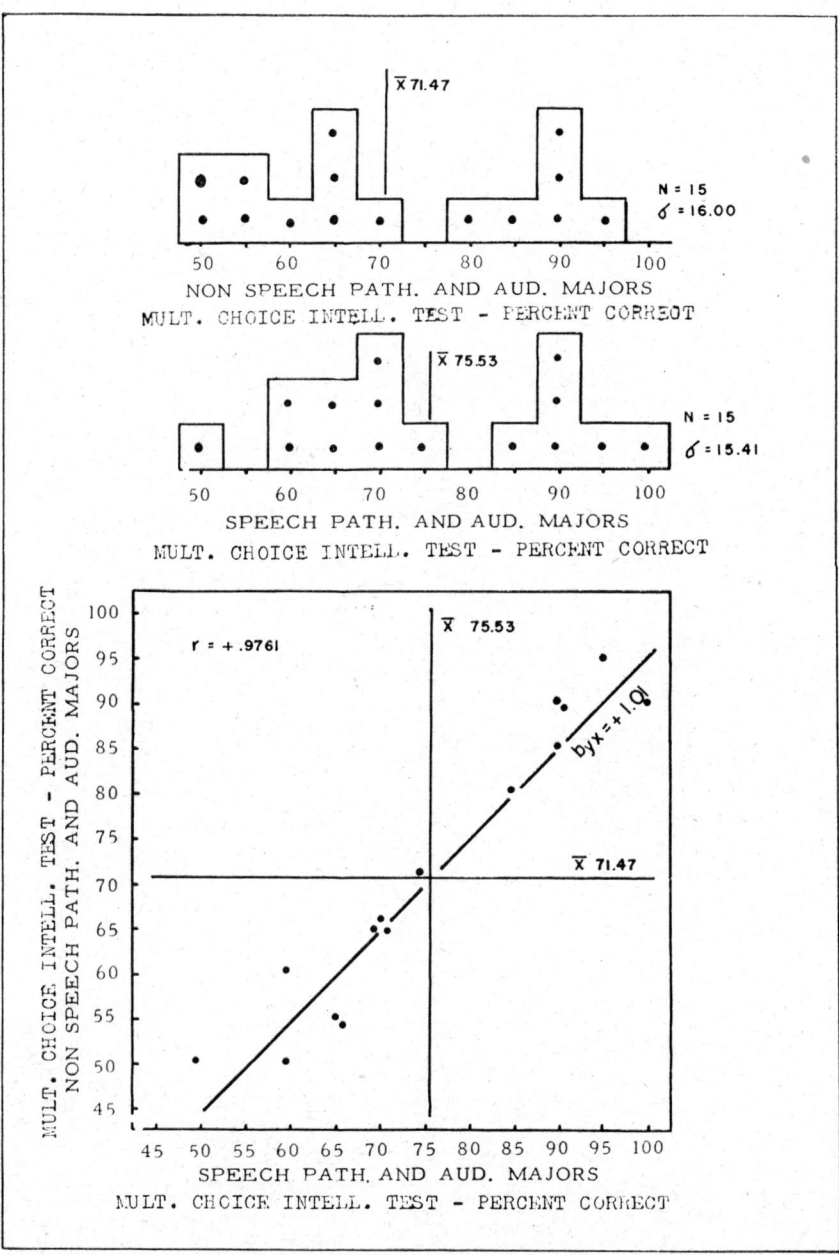

FIG. 29. Scatter diagram showing auditing scores of the speech pathology and audiology majors and the non-speech pathology and audiology majors on the multiple choice test in per cent correct in relation to the laryngectomized group, giving means, regression lines, and Pearson r, and also showing distributions of scores for the two auditing groups.

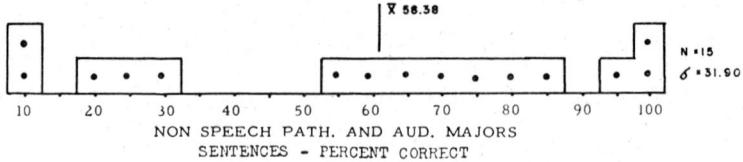

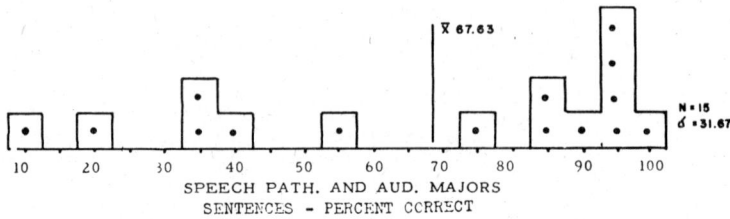

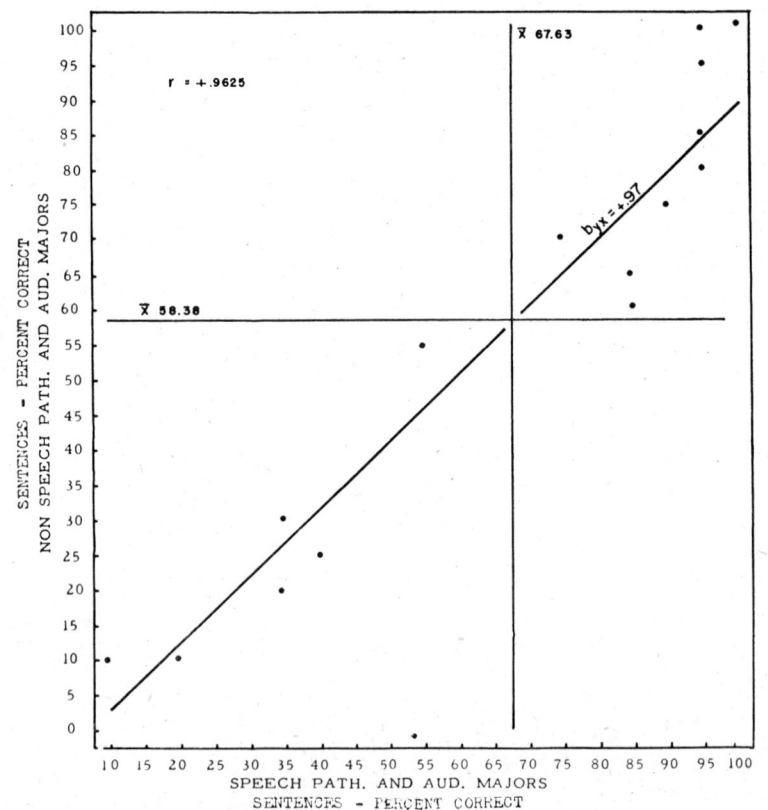

Fig. 30. Scatter diagram showing auditing scores of the speech pathology and audiology majors and the non-speech pathology and audiology majors on the sentences in per cent correct for the laryngectomized group, giving means, regression line, and Pearson r, and also showing distributions of scores for the two auditing groups.

INTELLIGIBILITY CRITERIA

Three intelligibility criteria were employed in this study in judging the intelligibility of the laryngectomized speakers. An attempt was made to select materials that would offer a variety of communication complexities. Figure 31 illustrates the ability of the three criteria to differentiate between laryngectomized speakers. Raw score distributions are indicated here.

The increasingly higher means from PB's to sentences, to multiple choice are illustrated. The sentences appear to discriminate between

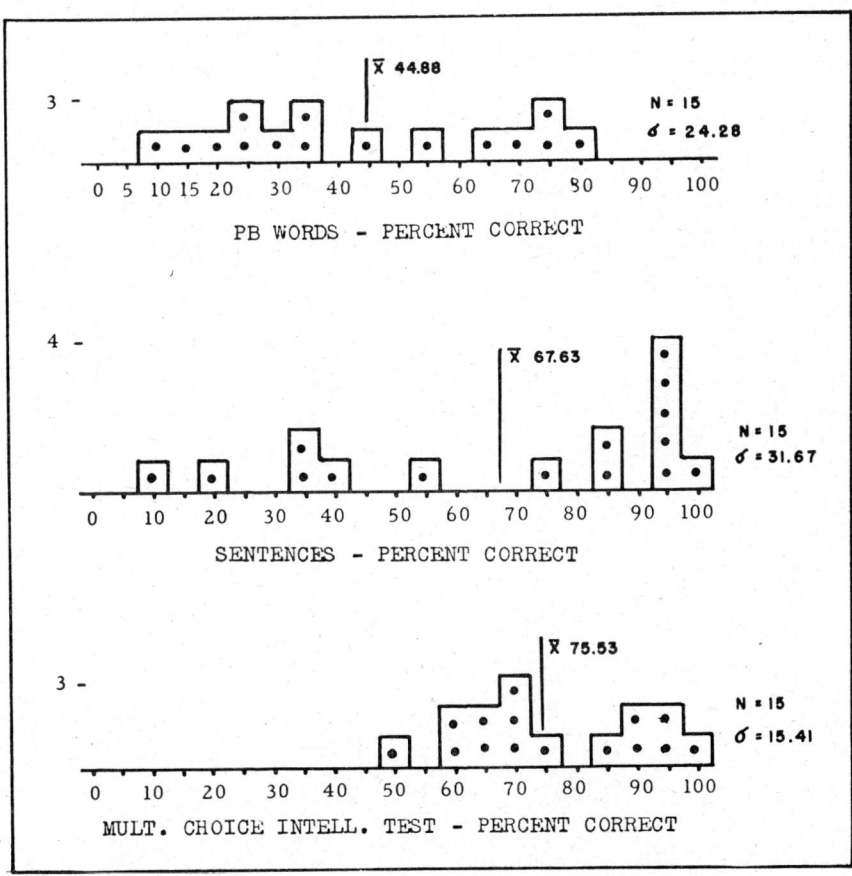

FIG. 31. Raw score distributions of the intelligibility of laryngectomized subjects on the three tests, PB's, sentences and multiple choice, showing x̄, N, and σ for each distribution.

speakers most adequately in terms of the actual spread of the distribution with scores in per cent correct ranging from below ten to one hundred. It is also observed that in the case of each criterion there appears to be a separate and distinct distribution of speakers below and above the mean.

The raw scores for each speaker on the three intelligibility tests were then converted into standard scores so as to allow for more legitimate comparisons between the three intelligibility criteria and between each laryngectomized speaker on the three tests.

Figure 32 indicates the distribution of standard scores for intelligibility on the three criteria. The subjects' numbers are indicated in the histogram. A combined $\bar{z}$ score separated the laryngectomized speakers into two distinct groups, one group above the $\bar{z}$ score mean, and one group below the $\bar{z}$ score mean. The $\bar{z}$ score distributions for the sentences, multiple choice and PB words are similar in that the division into two groups is observable but not as clearly marked. Although the speakers retain their relative position to each of the three distributions, some shifting is observable.

For this study the combined standard score grouping was considered to be a practical and justifiable manner of differentiating between the laryngectomized speakers on the basis of high and low intelligibility. The original raw scores for each intelligibility criteria, however, were utilized separately in computing the correlation data. The designation "high intelligibility" will be employed interchangeably for those individuals who fall within the $+\bar{z}$ group, and "low intelligibility" will be employed for those speakers who fall within the $-\bar{z}$ group. Table 11 summarizes the raw score and standard score data for each laryngectomized speaker on the three intelligibility tests, indicating the mean, standard deviation and variance for each test.

ARTICULATION ANALYSIS

PHONETIC AND ERROR ANALYSIS ACCORDING TO THE SOUND CATEGORIES

Phonetic analysis.–Table 12 presents the total number of occurrences of the sound categories for the 750 phonetically balanced monosyllabic words spoken by the laryngectomized individuals in this study. Of the total number of sounds, 1,609 are consonants, while 745 are vowels, comprising a total of 2,354 sounds. The consonant sounds are subdivided into nine categories; this classification was employed by Anderson (1) in his analysis of phonetically balanced monosyllabic words in his study.

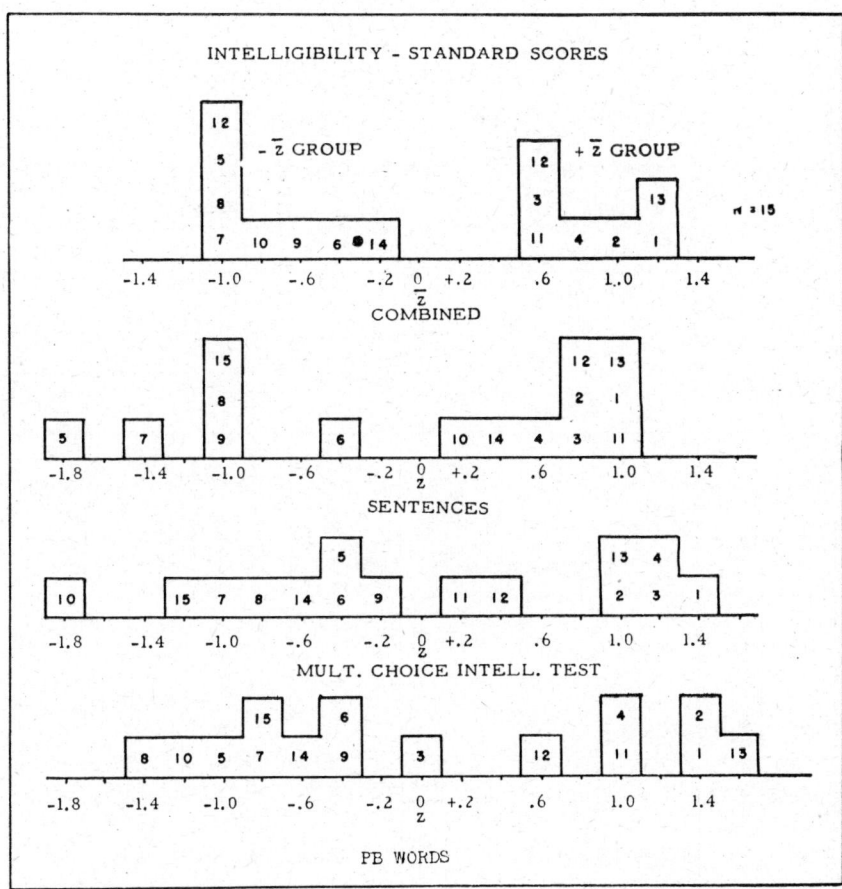

FIG. 32. Standard score distributions of the intelligibility of laryngectomized subjects on the three tests, sentences, multiple choice and PB words, showing the combined standard score distribution of the three intelligibility tests, which divides the scores into two groups, (1) those higher than the mean $+\bar{z}$ group and 2) those lower than the mean $-\bar{z}$ group. Numbers within figures correspond to the subject numbers (See Appendix, Table 53, p. 296).

Hyman (29) also used the same classification with some changes in the analysis of the sounds in his investigation. His speech samples were composed of constructed phonetically balanced monosyllabic nonsense material.

Table 13 compares the total number of the occurrences of the sounds in the various categories for the 750 phonetically balanced monosyllabic words spoken by the laryngectomized individuals in this study with the

TABLE 11

INTELLIGIBILITY RAW SCORES AND CORRESPONDING STANDARD SCORES FOR
EACH LARYNGECTOMIZED SPEAKER INCLUDING MEAN STANDARD SCORES
OF THREE INTELLIGIBILITY TESTS, PB LISTS, MULTIPLE CHOICE
TEST AND SENTENCES SHOWING MEANS, VARIANCES AND
STANDARD DEVIATIONS FOR EACH TEST

		PB		Multiple. Choice		Sentences		
$\bar{X}$		44.88		75.53		67.63		
σ^2		589.88		237.55		1,002.89		
σ		24.29		15.41		31.67		
Sub.	No.	Raw Score	Score	Raw Score	Score	Raw Score	Score	Mean Standard Score
P.S.	1	77.33	1.34	98	1.46	100	1.02	1.27
M.G.	2	77.00	1.32	92	1.07	93.12	.80	1.06
S.L.	3	43.60	- .05	94	1.20	93.33	.81	.65
L.J.	4	67.64	.94	93	1.13	84.50	.53	.87
R.C.M.	5	21.33	- .97	69	- .42	8.14	-1.88	-1.09
O.R.	6	34.00	- .45	70	- .36	56.00	- .37	- .39
J.K.	7	24.00	- .86	60	-1.01	21.89	-1.44	-1.10
C.K.	8	12.67	-1.33	64	- .75	37.71	- .94	-1.01
F.F.	9	36.00	- .37	72	- .23	35.60	-1.01	- .54
P.L.	10	18.00	-1.11	48	-1.79	75.33	.24	- .84
H.G.	11	66.80	.90	77	.10	96.11	.90	.63
F.M.	12	57.27	.51	83	.48	95.44	.88	.62
H.V.E.	13	82.83	1.56	90	.94	97.33	.94	1.15
G.B.	14	30.40	- .60	65	- .68	83.14	.49	- .26
M.A.	15	24.33	- .85	58	-1.14	36.89	- .97	- .99

materials used by Anderson's and Hyman's subjects. Analysis of the data shows a similarity between the consonant and vowel ratios for the three investigations.

Error analysis.—Table 14 indicates the error analysis for the 750 phonetically balanced monosyllabic words classified into the different sound categories and the percentages the sounds were incorrectly produced in the present investigation. A total of 501 sounds, or 357 consonants and 144 vowels, were incorrectly produced. The consonant errors are classified into voiced and voiceless categories. Of these sounds 200 fall into the voiced category while 157 fall into the voiceless category. The table indicates that 185 of the consonants are initial consonant errors while 122 are final consonant errors. Further breakdown reveals

TABLE 12

TOTAL NUMBER OF SOUNDS CLASSIFIED ACCORDING TO SOUND
CATEGORIES FOR 750 PHONETICALLY BALANCED MONOSYL-
LABIC WORDS SPOKEN BY THE LARYNGECTOMIZED
SPEAKERS IN THE PRESENT INVESTIGATION

Sound Categories	No. of Occurrences of Sounds
Consonants	1,609
Vowels	743
Total	2,354
Voiced consonants	867
Voiceless consonants	742
Initial consonants	697
Final consonants	696
Nasals	159
Stop plosives	742
Laterals	272
Fricatives	395
Glides	41
Total	1,609

that of the 357 consonant errors, 59 are nasals; 127, stop plosives; 39, laterals; 130, fricatives and 2, glides.

Table 15 presents the error analysis of the phonetically balanced monosyllabic materials classified according to sound categories produced incorrectly in the present investigation. When the error categories for the consonants are further broken down, of the 357 errors, 59 are nasals, 127 are stop plosives, 39 are laterals, 130 are fricatives and 2 are glides.

TABLE 13

TOTAL NUMBER OF THE OCCURRENCES OF SOUNDS CLASSIFIED
ACCORDING TO SOUND CATEGORIES FOR THE PHONETICALLY
BALANCED MONOSYLLABIC MATERIALS EMPLOYED
IN ANDERSON, HYMAN AND THE
PRESENT INVESTIGATION

Sound Categories	Anderson	Hyman	Present Investigation
Consonants	2,526	2,352	1,609
Vowels	1,218	896	745
Total			2,354
Voiced consonants	1,416	1,456	867
Voiceless consonants	1,224	896	742
Initial consonants	1,128	1,176	697
Final consonants	1,092	1,176	696
Nasals	420	280	159
Stop plosives	1,140	672	742
Laterals	344		272
Fricatives	632	840	395
Glides	87	336	41
Affricatives		224	
Total			1,609

Table 16 presents the number of times the sounds occur in their respective categories and the number and percentages of sounds in a category that were produced correctly in Anderson's, Hyman's and the
present investigation. Examination of Table 16 reveals that the consonants clustered in the various categories in a similar manner for the
three investigations. In the present investigation 1,252, or 78.8 per cent,
of a total of 1,609 consonants were produced correctly. Of 745 vowels,
601, or 80.7 per cent, were produced correctly. This would indicate that
in the present study the percentage of consonants and vowels produced

TABLE 14

ERROR ANALYSIS FOR 750 PHONETICALLY BALANCED MONOSYLLABIC
WORDS CLASSIFIED INTO THE DIFFERENT CATEGORIES
AND THE PERCENTAGES OF THE SOUNDS INCORRECTLY
PRODUCED IN THE PRESENT INVESTIGATION

Sound Categories	Present Investigation	
	Number	Percentage
Consonants	357	22.2
Vowels	144	19.3
Total	501	
Voiced consonants	200	23.1
Voiceless consonants	157	21.2
Initial consonants	185	26.5
Final consonants	122	17.5
Nasals	59	37.1
Stop plosives	127	17.1
Laterals	39	14.3
Fricatives	130	32.9
Glides	2	4.9
Total	357	

correctly are approximately equal. The ratio between the correct consonant and vowel production approaches one. This ratio contrasts
sharply with both Anderson's and Hyman's studies. Furthermore, the
three studies agree in terms of ratio for the correct production of voiced
and voiceless consonants. Further examination of the consonant categories reveals all the consonant sounds in all the categories in this study
were produced correctly more often than in either Anderson's or Hyman's studies with specific marked differences for the stop plosives,
laterals and glides. Examination of the table reveals that Anderson's
and Hyman's data for the consonant categories agree quite closely except
for the fricatives where the subjects in Anderson's study produced the

TABLE 15

ERROR ANALYSIS OF THE PHONETICALLY BALANCED MONOSYLLABIC
MATERIALS CLASSIFIED ACCORDING TO SOUND CATEGORIES
PRODUCED INCORRECTLY FOR ANDERSON, HYMAN AND
THE PRESENT INVESTIGATION

Sound Categories	Anderson	Hyman	Present Investigation
Consonants	1,377	1,430	357
Vowels	486	310	144
Total			501
Voiced consonants	731	839	200
Voiceless consonants	710	591	157
Initial consonants	588	696	185
Final consonants	627	734	122
Nasals	208	146	59
Stop plosives	631	382	127
Laterals	162		39
Fricatives	369	631	130
Glides	43	163	2
Affricatives		106	
Total			357

fricatives correctly approximately twice as often as in Hyman's study.
Figure 33 presents these relationships of correctly produced sounds in
their respective consonant and vowel categories.

Table 17 shows the sound categories listed from most to least intelligible according to the percentages of sounds in the various categories produced correctly in Anderson's, Hyman's and the present investigation.
In Anderson's and Hyman's studies the vowels are ranked as most often
correctly produced. The present investigation ranks the vowels fifth;
although with the exception of the glides the percentages for the next
five categories are quite similar. The final consonant category is ranked

TABLE 16

THE NUMBER OF THE SOUNDS OCCURRING IN THEIR RESPECTIVE CATEGORIES AND THE
NUMBER AND PERCENTAGES OF SOUNDS IN VARIOUS CATEGORIES PRODUCED COR-
RECTLY FOR PHONETICALLY BALANCED MONOSYLLABIC MATERIALS IN
ANDERSON'S, HYMAN'S AND THE PRESENT INVESTIGATION

Sound Categories	Number of Times Sounds Occurred			Number and Percentage of Times Sounds Produced Correctly					
	Anderson	Hyman	Present Invest.	Anderson		Hyman		Present Invest.	
	Number	Number	Number	Num-ber	Per-cent	Num-ber	Per-cent	Num-ber	Per-cent
Consonants	2,526	2,352	1,609	1,149	45.48	922	39.20	1,252	77.8
Vowels	1,218	896	745	732	60.09	586	65.40	601	80.7
Total number sounds	3,744	3,248	2,354	1,881		1,508		1,852	
Voiced consonants	1,416	1,456	867	685	48.37	617	42.38	667	76.9
Voiceless consonants	1,224	896	742	514	41.99	305	34.04	585	78.8
Initial consonants	1,128	1,176	697	540	47.87	480	40.82	512	73.5
Final consonants	1,092	1,176	696	465	42.50	442	37.58	574	82.5
Nasals	420	280	159	212	50.47	134	47.86	100	62.9
Stop plosives	1,140	672	742	509	44.64	290	43.15	615	82.9
Laterals	344		272	182	52.90			233	85.7
Fricatives	632	840	395	263	41.61	209	24.99	265	67.1
Glides	87	336	41	44	50.57	171	50.89	39	95.1
Affricatives		224				118			
Total number conso-nants occurring	2,526	2,352	1,609	1,210		922		1,252	

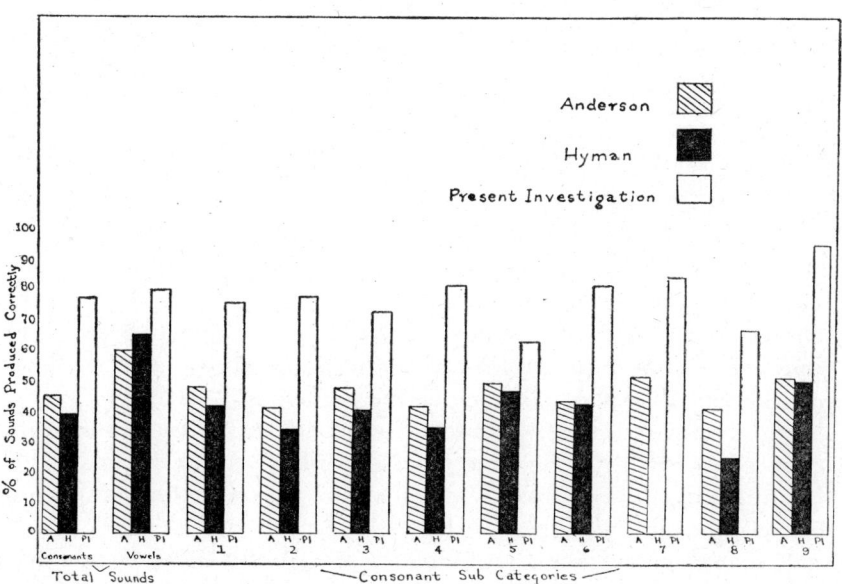

FIG. 33. Percentages of sounds produced correctly in the various consonant
and vowel categories in Anderson's, Hyman's and the present investigation
for phonetically balanced materials. Categories: 1) total consonants, 2) total
vowels. Consonant sub categories: 1) voiced, 2) voiceless, 3) initial, 4) final,
5) nasals, 6) stop plosives, 78) laterals, 8) fricatives, 9) glides.

TABLE 17

SOUND CATEGORIES LISTED FROM MOST TO LEAST INTELLIGIBLE ACCORDING TO
THE PERCENTAGES OF THE SOUNDS IN THE VARIOUS CATEGORIES
PRODUCED CORRECTLY IN ANDERSON'S, HYMAN'S
AND THE PRESENT INVESTIGATION

Anderson		Hyman		Present Investigation	
Sound Categories	Percent	Sound Categories	Percent	Sound Categories	Percent
Vowels	60.09	Vowels	65.40	Glides	95.1
Laterals	52.90	Affricatives	52.68	Laterals	85.7
Glides	50.57	Glides	50.89	Stop plosives	82.9
Nasals	50.47	Nasals	47.86	Final consonants	82.5
Voiced consonants	48.37	Stop plosives	43.15	Vowels	80.7
Initial consonants	47.87	Voiced consonants	42.38	Voiceless consonants	78.8
Stop plosives	44.64	Initial consonants	40.82	Voiced consonants	76.9
Final consonants	42.50	Final consonants	37.58	Initial consonants	73.5
Voiceless consonants	41.99	Voiceless consonants	34.04	Fricatives	67.2
Fricatives	41.61	Fricatives	24.88	Nasals	62.9

eighth by Anderson and Hyman, while in the present investigation the final consonant category is ranked fourth. The nasals are ranked fourth by Anderson and Hyman, while they are ranked tenth in the present investigation, indicating that for the individuals in this study the nasal sounds were the most difficult for the subjects to produce. The three studies agree closely with respect to the production of the fricative sounds.

PHONETIC AND ERROR ANALYSIS FOR THE HIGH AND LOW INTELLIGIBILITY LARYNGECTOMIZED SPEAKERS

Phonetic analysis.—Table 18 presents the phonetic analysis for the phonetically balanced words for the high and low intelligibility groups according to Anderson's and Hyman's sound classifications and the percentages of occurrence of sounds in each category. The table reveals an expected relationship since the phonetically balanced material is approximately divided equally among the two groups.

Error analysis.—Table 19 shows the error analysis of the phonetically balanced words of the high and low intelligibility speakers classified in the different sound categories and the percentages of incorrectly produced sounds in the different categories. Inspection of the data also reveals that in every category the high intelligibility speakers produced fewer errors. Inspection of the data also reveals that the nasals were produced incorrectly 3.9 per cent for the high intelligibility speakers as against 67.5 per cent for the low intelligibility speakers. This difference is also marked in the fricatives where the proportion of errors is twice as great for the low intelligibility speakers.

TABLE 18

PHONETIC ANALYSIS OF THE PHONETICALLY BALANCED WORDS FOR
HIGH AND LOW INTELLIGIBILITY GROUPS OF THE PRESENT
INVESTIGATION ACCORDING TO SOUND CATEGORIES,
CLASSIFICATION AND PERCENTAGES OF OCCUR-
RENCE OF SOUNDS IN EACH CATEGORY FOR
THE SEVEN HIGH INTELLIGIBILITY
AND EIGHT LOW INTELLIGIBILITY
LARYNGECTOMIZED SPEAKERS

Sound Categories	High Intelligibility		Low Intelligibility	
	Number	Percent	Number	Percent
Consonants	743	68.4	866	68.3
Vowels	343	31.6	402	31.7
Total sounds	1,086		1,268	
Voiced consonants	400	53.8	467	53.9
Voiceless consonants	343	46.2	399	46.1
Initial consonants	326	43.9	371	42.8
Final consonants	326	43.9	370	42.7
Nasals	76	10.2	83	9.6
Stop plosives	317	42.7	425	49.1
Laterals	126	17.0	146	16.9
Fricatives	206	27.7	189	21.8
Glides	18	2.4	23	2.7
Total consonants	743		866	

Table 20 shows the same relationship in terms of the sounds produced
correctly in the various consonant and vowel categories. This data reveals that the high intelligibility speakers produced all the sounds in
every category correctly more often than the low intelligibility speakers.
Figure 34 illustrates these relationships.

Table 21 indicates the sound categories listed from most to least intelligible according to the percentages of sounds in the various categories produced correctly for the seven high and eight low intelligibility

TABLE 19

ERROR ANALYSIS OF THE PHONETICALLY BALANCED WORDS FOR THE HIGH
AND LOW INTELLIGIBILITY GROUPS OF THE PRESENT INVESTIGATION
ACCORDING TO SOUND CATEGORIES CLASSIFICATION AND THE
PERCENTAGES OF OCCURRENCE OF SOUNDS IN EACH CATE-
GORY FOR THE SEVEN HIGH INTELLIGIBILITY
AND EIGHT LOW INTELLIGIBILITY
LARYNGECTOMIZED SPEAKERS

Sound Categories	High Intelligibility		Low Intelligibility	
	Number of Errors	Percent of Sounds	Number of Errors	Percent of Sounds
Consonants	51	6.9	306	35.3
Vowels	24	7.0	120	29.8
Total	75		426	
Voiced consonants	20	5.0	165	35.3
Voiceless consonants	31	9.0	141	35.3
Initial consonants	31	9.5	154	41.5
Final consonants	13	4.0	109	29.5
Nasals	3	3.9	56	67.3
Stop plosives	15	4.7	112	26.3
Laterals	9	7.1	30	20.5
Fricatives	24	11.6	106	56.1
Glides	0	0.0	2	8.7
Total	51		306	

speakers. Examination of the data reveals that the percentages and the
ranking for the total group are markedly similar to those for the low intelligibility group, while the percentages and ranking for the high intelligibility group show differences between the high and low intelligibility speakers. For example, the nasals are ranked second with a 96.1
per cent correct production for the high intelligibility speakers, while
the same category ranks tenth with a 32.5 per cent correct production for
the low intelligibility speakers. The nasal category is also ranked tenth
for the total group. This would indicate that the performance of the low

intelligibility speakers contributes a large weighting to the percentages of the entire group. Figure 35 shows these relationships.

TABLE 20

THE NUMBER AND PERCENTAGES OF SOUNDS OCCURRING IN THEIR RESPECTIVE CATEGORIES
AND THE NUMBER AND PERCENTAGES OF SOUNDS IN THE VARIOUS CATEGORIES
PRODUCED CORRECTLY FOR THE SEVEN HIGH AND EIGHT LOW
INTELLIGIBILITY LARYNGECTOMIZED SPEAKERS
IN PB WORDS

Sound Categories	Number and Percentage of Times Sound Category Occurred				Number and Percentage of Times Sound Category Produced Correctly			
	High		Low		High		Low	
	Number	Percent	Number	Percent	Number	Percent	Number	Percent
Consonants	743	68.4	866	68.3	692	93.1	560	64.7
Vowels	343	31.6	402	31.7	319	93.0	282	70.2
Total number of sounds	1,086		1,268					
Voiced consonants	400	53.8	467	53.9	380	95.0	302	64.7
Voiceless consonants	343	46.2	399	46.1	312	91.0	258	64.7
Initial consonants	326	43.9	371	42.8	295	90.5	217	58.5
Final consonants	326	43.9	370	42.7	313	96.0	261	70.5
Nasals	76	10.2	83	9.6	73	96.1	27	32.5
Stop plosives	317	42.7	425	49.1	302	95.3	313	73.7
Laterals	126	17.0	146	17.9	117	92.9	116	79.5
Fricatives	206	27.7	189	21.8	182	88.4	83	43.9
Glides	18	2.4	23	2.7	18	100	21	91.3
Total number of consonants occurring	743		866					

TABLE 21

SOUND CATEGORIES LISTED FROM MOST TO LEAST INTELLIGIBLE ACCORDING TO THE
PERCENTAGES OF SOUNDS IN THE VARIOUS CATEGORIES PRODUCED CORRECTLY
FOR THE SEVEN HIGH INTELLIGIBILITY AND EIGHT LOW
INTELLIGIBILITY SPEAKERS IN PB WORDS

High Intelligibility		Low Intelligibility		Total Laryngectomy Group	
Sound Categories	Percent of Sounds Produced Correctly	Sound Categories	Percent of Sounds Produced Correctly	Sound Categories	Percent of Sounds Produced Correctly
Glides	100	Glides	91.3	Glides	95.1
Nasals	96.1	Laterals	79.5	Laterals	85.7
Final consonants	96.0	Stop plosives	73.7	Stop plosives	82.9
Stop plosives	95.3	Final consonants	70.5	Final consonants	82.5
Voiced consonants	95.0	Vowels	70.2	Vowels	80.7
Vowels	93.0	Voiced consonants	64.7	Voiceless consonants	78.8
Laterals	92.9	Voiceless consonants	64.7	Voiced consonants	76.9
Voiceless consonants	91.0	Initial consonants	58.5	Initial consonants	73.
Initial consonants	90.5	Fricatives	43.9	Fricatives	67.1
Fricatives	88.4	Nasals	32.5	Nasals	62.9

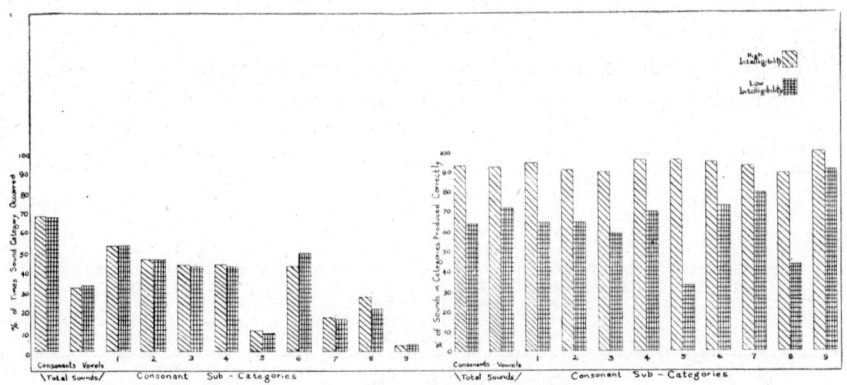

FIG. 34. Percentages of sounds occurring in the various consonant and vowel categories and the percentages of sounds produced correctly in these categories for the seven high and eight low intelligibility laryngectomized speakers for PB words. Categories: 1) total consonants, 2) total vowels. Consonant sub categories: 1) voiced, 2) voiceless, 3) initial, 4) final, 5) nasals, 6) stop plosives, 7) laterals, 8) fricatives, 9) glides.

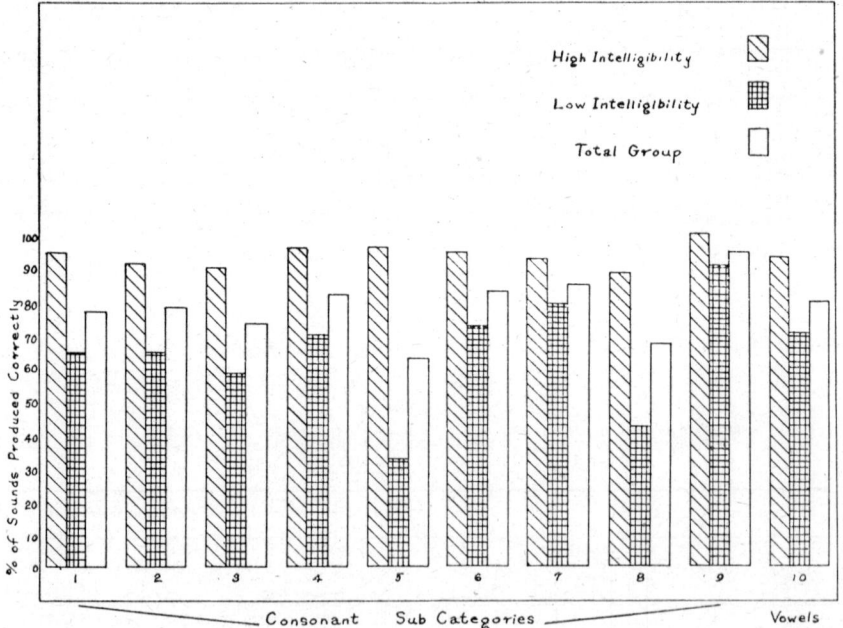

FIG. 35. Percentages of sounds produced correctly in the various consonant and vowel categories for the seven high and eight low intelligibility laryngectomized speakers and for the total group for PB words. Sound categories: 1) voiced consonants, 2) voiceless consonants, 3) initial consonants, 4) final consonants, 5) nasal consonants, 6) stop plosive consonants, 7) lateral consonants, 8) fricative consonants, 9) glide consonants, 10) vowels.

PHONETIC AND ERROR ANALYSIS ACCORDING TO THE VARIOUS ERROR CATEGORIES

The preceding analysis has been based upon sound categories established by Anderson and Hyman in their investigations. Anderson and Hyman employ a general sound classification system which permits consideration of errors in a certain sound category but does not provide information relative to the type of errors occurring within the various error categories. It would therefore seem desirable to utilize a system which would permit analysis of the different types of errors. Hudgins (23) has used such a system in his investigation of the speech intelligibility of the deaf.

TABLE 22

TOTAL NUMBER OF POSSIBLE ERRORS CLASSIFIED ACCORDING
TO SOUND ERROR CATEGORIES FOR 150 SENTENCES AND
750 PHONETICALLY BALANCED MONOSYLLABIC WORDS
SPOKEN BY THE LARYNGECTOMIZED SPEAKERS
IN THE PRESENT INVESTIGATION

	Error Categories	Number of Possible Errors	
		Sentences	PB Words
Consonants	Surd-sonant	771	796
	Substitution	1,496	1,370
	Compound consonants	240	261
	Releasing consonants	749	550
	Arresting consonants	460	526
	Constructive compound	1,496	1,370
	Total	1,496	1,370
Vowels	Substitution	1,063	745
	Diphtongization	859	527
	Neutralization	1,063	745
	Omission	1,063	745
	Constructive release	1,063	745
	Total	1,063	745

Phonetic analysis.—Table 22 indicates the number of possible errors for both sentence and PB materials for the different error categories. The sentences provide opportunity for a total of 1,496 possible consonant errors, while the PB materials provide opportunity for a total of 1,370 possible consonant errors. The breakdown of the sentences and the PB materials into the various error categories reveals a proportional distribution of the sounds for both the sentences and the PB materials. Table 22 also indicates the total number of possible vowel errors for both types of materials.

Error analysis.—Table 23 presents the error analysis for 150 sentences and 750 phonetically balanced monosyllabic words classified into the different error categories and the percentages of the sounds incorrectly produced in the present investigation. The table indicates that for the

TABLE 23

ERROR ANALYSIS FOR 150 SENTENCES AND 750 PHONETICALLY BALANCED
MONOSYLLABIC WORDS CLASSIFIED INTO THE DIFFERENT ERROR
CATEGORIES AND THE PERCENTAGES OF THE SOUNDS
INCORRECTLY PRODUCED IN THE
PRESENT INVESTIGATION

Error Categories	Sentences		PB Words	
	Number of Errors	Percent of Sounds Incorrectly Produced	Number of Errors	Percent of Sounds Incorrectly Produced
Consonants				
Surd-sonant	40	5.2	86	10.8
Substitution	113	7.6	175	12.8
Compound consonants	36	15.0	33	12.6
Releasing consonants	96	12.8	27	4.9
Arresting consonants	74	16.1	18	3.5
Constructive compound	38	2.5	46	3.4
Vowels				
Substitution	20	1.9	55	10.4
Diphthongization	4	.4	24	4.6
Neutralization	7	.8	48	9.1
Omission	31	2.4	0	0
Constructive release	33	3.1	20	3.5

consonants the substitution error category contains the greatest number of errors for both the sentences and the PB materials. The table also reveals that the releasing and arresting consonants were incorrectly spoken approximately four times as often for the sentences as for the PB materials. Furthermore, the vowel error categories for the PB's show a greater over-all number of errors than for the vowels in the sentence materials.

Table 24 shows the number of possible errors and the number and percentages of correct sounds in the various categories. This table indicates that with the exception of the releasing and arresting consonant error categories, no marked differences exist for sentences and PB materials. Percentages indicate the releasing and arresting consonants were produced correctly more often for the PB than for the sentence material. Figure 36 illustrates the percentages of correctly produced consonants and vowels in their proper categories for the sentences. Figure 37 shows

TABLE 24

THE NUMBER OF POSSIBLE ERRORS AND THE NUMBER AND
PERCENTAGES OF CORRECT SOUNDS IN THE VARIOUS
CATEGORIES FOR SENTENCES AND PB WORDS
IN THE PRESENT INVESTIGATION

	Error Categories	Number of Possible Errors		Number of Correct Sounds		Percent of Correct Sounds	
		Sentences	PB	Sentences	PB	Sentences	PB
Consonants	Surd-sonant	771	795	731	709	94.8	89.2
	Substitution	1,496	1,370	1,383	1,195	92.4	87.2
	Compound consonants	240	261	204	228	85.0	87.4
	Releasing consonants	749	550	653	523	87.2	95.1
	Arresting consonants	460	526	386	508	83.9	96.5
	Constructive compound	1,496	1,370	1,458	1,324	97.5	96.6
Vowels	Substitution	1,063	745	1,043	690	98.1	92.6
	Diphthongization	859	527	855	503	98.3	95.4
	Neutralization	1,063	745	1,056	697	99.2	93.5
	Omission	1,063	745	1,032	745	97.6	100
	Constructive release	1,063	745	1,030	725	96.9	97.3

the percentages of correctly produced consonants and vowels in their proper categories for the PB materials.

Table 25 shows a ranking of the vowel and consonant categories according to the percentages of sounds correctly produced for the 150 sentences and the 750 phonetically balanced monosyllabic words for the present study. The table indicates that for the sentences the vowel categories have a greater percentage of correctly produced sounds, while this relationship does not hold for the PB words. The releasing compound and arresting consonants have the smallest percentage of correct production for the sentence material. The arresting and releasing consonants were produced correctly more often in the PB material than for the sentences, while the compound consonants are ranked the same for both. Figure 38 illustrates these relationships.

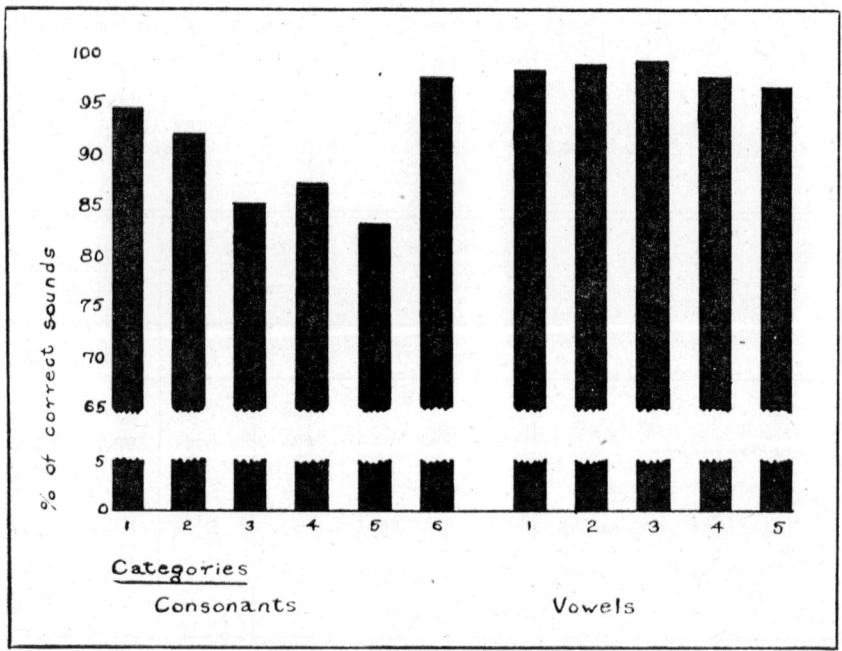

Fig. 36. Percentages of sounds produced correctly in the various consonant and vowel error categories for the fifteen laryngectomized speakers for the sentences.
Consonant error categories: 1) surd-sonant, 2) substitution, 3) compound consonant, 4) releasing consonant, 5) arresting consonant, 6) constructive compound.
Vowel error categories: 1) substitution, 2) diphthongization, 3) neutralization, 4) omission, 5) constructive release.

PHONETIC AND ERROR ANALYSIS FOR THE HIGH AND LOW INTELLIGIBILITY
LARYNGECTOMIZED SPEAKERS

Phonetic analysis.—Table 26 shows the total number of possible errors
classified according to sound error categories for 150 sentences and 750
PB monosyllabic words spoken by the seven high and eight low intelligibility laryngectomized speakers in the present investigation. The
clusters of sounds for both the sentence and PB materials appear to be
more or less equally distributed.

Error analysis.—Table 27 presents the error analysis for the 150 sentences and the 750 phonetically balanced monosyllabic words classified
into the different error categories for the seven high and eight low intelligibility laryngectomized speakers. Examination of the table reveals

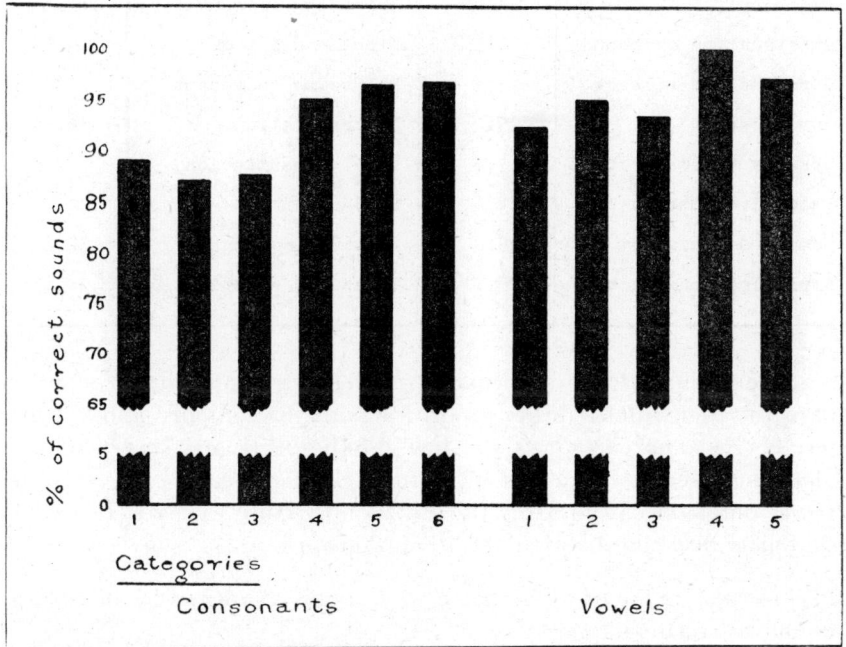

FIG. 37. Percentages of sounds produced correctly in the various consonant
and vowel error categories for the fifteen laryngectomized speakers for the
PB words.
Consonant error categories: 1) surd-sonant, 2) substitution, 3) compound
consonant, 4) releasing consonant, 5) arresting consonant, 6) constructive
compound.
Vowel error categories: 1) substitution, 2) diphthongization, 3) neutralization, 4) omission, 5) constructive release.

TABLE 25

RANKING OF THE VOWEL AND CONSONANT CATEGORIES ACCORDING TO THE
PERCENTAGES OF SOUNDS INCORRECTLY PRODUCED FOR THE 150
SENTENCES AND THE 750 PHONETICALLY BALANCED
MONOSYLLABIC WORDS IN THE PRESENT
INVESTIGATION

Sentences		PB Words	
Error Categories	Percent of Errors	Error Categories	Percent of Errors
Neutralization	.8	Omission	0
Diphthongization	1.7	Constructive release	2.7
Vowel substitution	1.9	Constructive compound	3.4
Omission	2.4	Arresting consonant	3.5
Constructive compound	2.5	Diphthongization	4.6
Constructive release	3.1	Releasing consonant	4.9
Surd-sonant	5.2	Neutralization	6.5
Consonant substitution	7.6	Vowel substitution	7.4
Releasing consonant	12.8	Surd-sonant	10.8
Compound consonant	15.0	Compound consonant	12.6
Arresting consonants	16.1	Consonant substitution	12.8

that the low intelligibility speakers produced a greater number of errors
than the high intelligibility group for both the sentence and PB materials. In some categories the low intelligibility speakers produced
many more errors than the high intelligibility speakers. In only the
vowel omission category for the PB monosyllabic words is there any
similarity between the high and the low groups.

PERCENTAGE OF SOUNDS AND ERROR CATEGORIES AND RANKING OF SOUNDS
IN ORDER OF DIFFICULTY

Table 28 presents the consonant sounds ranked according to difficulty,
occurrence of sounds, percentage of occurrence of each sound, number
of errors for each sound and percentage of errors for each sound for the
150 sentences spoken by the fifteen laryngectomized individuals. The
unvoiced [θ] and [h] were spoken proportionately more times incorrectly than any other sounds. The [θ] was spoken incorrectly every time it
was produced while the [h] sound was spoken incorrectly 97 per cent of

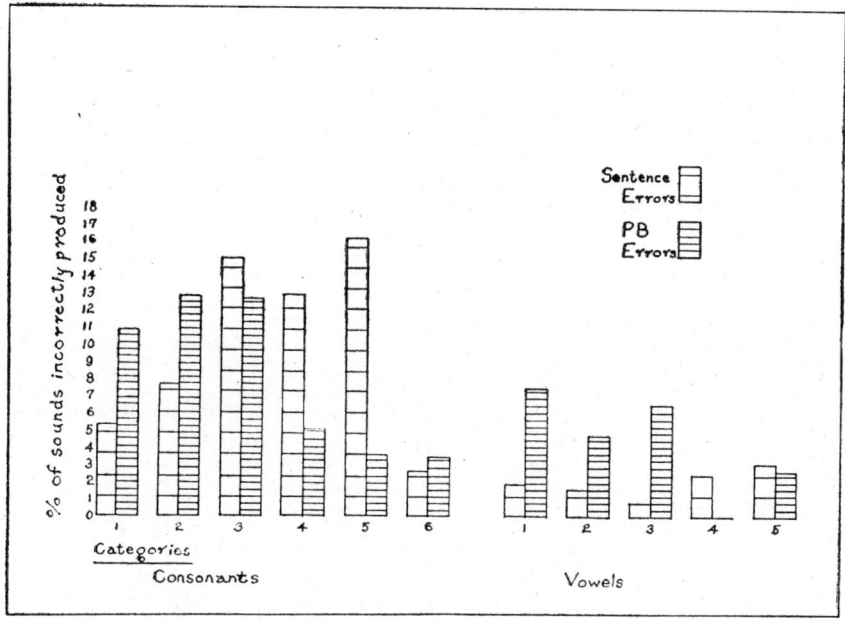

FIG. 38. Percentages of sounds produced incorrectly in the various consonant and vowel error categories for the 150 sentences and 750 phonetically balanced monosyllabic words.

Consonant error categories: 1) surd-sonant, 2) substitution, 3) compound consonant, 4) releasing consonant, 5) arresting consonant, 6) constructive compound.

Vowel error categories: 1) substitution, 2) diphthongization, 3) neutralization, 4) omission, 5) constructive release.

the time. The next sound ranked according to difficulty is the [ð]. It was spoken incorrectly 64.3 per cent of the time. This would indicate that the [h] sound was spoken incorrectly nine times out of ten. The [ð] was spoken incorrectly six times out of ten. The next sound in order of difficulty is the [d]. This was spoken 38.4 per cent incorrectly or approximately four out of ten times; [j] and [l] appear to have the same degree of difficulty, since errors were made approximately three out of ten times. The next six sounds [v], [r], [p], [w], [ŋ] and [f], appear to have about the same difficulty, since they were spoken incorrectly two or three times out of ten; while the remaining sounds were spoken two or less times out of ten.

Tables 29 and 30 show the consonant sounds ranked according to difficulty, occurrence of sounds, percentage of occurrence of each sound, number of errors for each sound and percentage of errors for each sound for the 150 sentences spoken by the seven high and eight low intelligibility laryngectomized speakers. These tables indicate that for both the high and low groups the same three sounds which were difficult for the total group maintain the same ranking excepting that [ð] was spoken incorrectly 52 per cent of the time for the high group, while it was spoken incorrectly 76.5 per cent of the time for the low group. Examination of the table also reveals that a change of ranks takes place in the consonants

TABLE 26

TOTAL NUMBER OF POSSIBLE ERRORS OF SOUNDS CLASSIFIED ACCORD-
ING TO ERROR CATEGORIES FOR 150 SENTENCES AND 750
PHONETICALLY BALANCED MONOSYLLABIC WORDS SPOKEN
BY THE SEVEN HIGH INTELLIGIBILITY AND EIGHT
LOW INTELLIGIBILITY LARYNGECTOMIZED
SPEAKERS IN THE PRESENT
INVESTIGATION

Error Categories	Number of Possible Errors			
	Sentences		PB Words	
	High	Low	High	Low
Consonants				
Surd-sonant	357	414	377	418
Substitution	706	790	636	734
Compound consonants	123	117	120	141
Releasing consonants	310	439	239	291
Arresting consonants	233	227	236	290
Constructive compound	706	790	636	734
Vowels				
Substitution	487	576	343	402
Diphthongization	387	472	238	289
Neutralization	487	576	343	402
Omission	487	576	343	402
Constructive release	487	576	343	402

after the first three sounds between the high and low groups and that the low group produced every sound except [ʒ] and [ʍ] incorrectly more often than the high group. Twenty-two sounds of the twenty-five for the high group were spoken incorrectly two or less times out of ten, while for the low group twelve sounds were spoken incorrectly two or less times out of ten.

Table 31 shows the consonant sounds ranked according to difficulty, occurrence of sounds, percentage of occurrence of each sound, number

TABLE 27

ERROR ANALYSIS FOR 150 SENTENCES AND 750 PHONETICALLY
BALANCED MONOSYLLABIC WORDS CLASSIFIED INTO THE
DIFFERENT ERROR CATEGORIES FOR THE SEVEN HIGH
AND EIGHT LOW INTELLIGIBILITY LARYNGECTOMIZED
SPEAKERS IN THE PRESENT
INVESTIGATION

	Error Categories	Sentences			PB Words		
		High	Low	Total	High	Low	Total
Consonants	Surd-sonant	7	33	40	11	75	86
	Substitution	42	71	113	32	143	175
	Compound consonants	10	26	36	6	27	33
	Releasing consonants	25	71	96	11	16	27
	Arresting consonants	7	67	74	1	17	18
	Constructive compound	16	22	38	6	40	46
	Total	107	290	397	67	318	385
Vowels	Substitution	3	17	20	13	42	55
	Diphthongization	2	2	4	6	18	24
	Neutralization	0	7	7	4	44	48
	Omission	0	31	31	0	0	0
	Constructive release	6	27	33	4	16	20
	Total	11	84	95	27	120	147

of errors for each sound and the percentage of errors for each sound for
the 750 PB words spoken by the total group of laryngectomized speakers.
Inspection of the table shows that [ʍ] and [j] were misarticulated every
time they were produced and that [h] was incorrectly produced 97 per
cent of the time; [ð] and [ʒ] were produced incorrectly 50 per cent of the
time, while [n] and [z] were produced on the average of four out of every

TABLE 28

CONSONANT SOUNDS RANKED ACCORDING TO DIFFICULTY, OCCURRENCE
OF SOUNDS, PERCENTAGE OF OCCURRENCE OF EACH SOUND, NUMBER
OF ERRORS FOR EACH SOUND AND PERCENTAGE OF ERRORS FOR
EACH SOUND FOR THE 150 SENTENCES SPOKEN BY THE
FIFTEEN LARYNGECTOMIZED SPEAKERS

Sounds Ranked in Order of Difficulty	Occurrence of Sounds	Percent of Occurrence of Sounds	Number of Errors for Sounds	Percent of Errors of Sounds
[θ]	5	.4	5	100
[h]	69	5.5	67	97.1
[ð]	171	13.6	110	64.3
[d]	73	5.8	28	38.4
[j]	6	.5	2	33.3
[l]	59	4.7	19	32.2
[v]	28	2.2	8	29.1
[r]	90	7.2	26	28.9
[p]	39	3.1	11	28.2
[w]	71	5.6	18	25.4
[ŋ]	21	1.7	5	23.8
[f]	40	3.2	9	22.5
[m]	45	3.6	9	20.0
[k]	58	4.6	11	19.0
[ʃ]	27	2.1	5	18.5
[g]	11	.9	2	18.2
[n]	124	9.9	20	16.1
[t]	118	9.4	17	14.4
[s]	56	4.5	7	12.5
[dʒ]	16	1.3	2	12.5
[tʃ]	19	1.5	2	10.5
[b]	40	3.2	4	10.0
[z]	65	5.2	4	6.2
[ʒ]	2	.2	0	0
[ʍ]	4	.3	0	0

ten times incorrectly. The next five sounds were produced three out of
ten times incorrectly, while the remaining sounds were produced incorrectly two or less times out of every ten times uttered.

Table 32 presents the consonant sounds ranked according to difficulty,
occurrence of sounds, percentages of occurrence of each sound, number
of errors for sounds and the percentage of errors for each sound for the

TABLE 29

CONSONANT SOUNDS RANKED ACCORDING TO DIFFICULTY, OCCURRENCE
OF SOUNDS, PERCENTAGE OF OCCURRENCE OF EACH SOUND, NUMBER
OF ERRORS FOR EACH SOUND AND PERCENTAGE OF ERRORS FOR
EACH SOUND FOR THE 150 SENTENCES SPOKEN BY THE
SEVEN HIGH INTELLIGIBILITY
LARYNGECTOMIZED SPEAKERS

Sounds Ranked in Order of Difficulty	Occurrence of Sounds	Percent of Occurrence of Sounds	Number of Errors for Sounds	Percent of Errors of Sounds
[θ]	1	.2	1	100
[h]	26	4.5	24	92.3
[ð]	86	14.8	45	52.3
[g]	4	.7	1	25.0
[j]	4	.7	1	25.0
[p]	18	3.1	4	22.2
[f]	19	3.3	4	21.1
[t]	51	8.8	8	15.7
[d]	32	5.5	4	12.5
[k]	24	4.1	3	12.5
[ʃ]	16	2.8	2	12.5
[r]	37	6.4	4	10.8
[v]	10	1.7	1	10.0
[l]	26	4.5	2	7.7
[s]	23	4.0	1	4.3
[w]	33	5.7	1	3.0
[n]	67	11.6	1	1.5
[b]	18	3.1	0	0
[z]	33	5.7	0	0
[ʒ]	1	.2	0	0
[tʃ]	9	1.6	0	0
[dʒ]	9	1.6	0	0
[ʍ]	2	3.4	0	0
[m]	19	3.3	0	0
[ŋ]	12	2.1	0	0

750 PB words spoken by the seven high and eight low intelligibility laryngectomized speakers. In this instance the [h] and [ʍ] were produced incorrectly every time the sound appeared. All of the remaining sounds were produced two or less times out of ten incorrectly; while in Table 33 the relationship for the group is much different. Here all sounds but five were produced three or more times incorrectly out of every ten times.

TABLE 30

CONSONANT SOUNDS RANKED ACCORDING TO DIFFICULTY, OCCURRENCE
OF SOUNDS, PERCENTAGE OF OCCURRENCE OF EACH SOUND, NUMBER
OF ERRORS FOR EACH SOUND AND PERCENTAGE OF ERRORS FOR
EACH SOUND FOR THE 150 SENTENCES SPOKEN BY THE
EIGHT LOW INTELLIGIBILITY
LARYNGECTOMIZED SPEAKERS

Sounds Ranked in Order of Difficulty	Occurrence of Sounds	Percent of Occurrence of Sounds	Number of Errors for Sounds	Percent of Errors of Sounds
[θ]	4	.6	4	100
[h]	43	6.4	43	100
[ð]	85	12.6	65	76.5
[d]	41	6.1	24	58.5
[ŋ]	9	1.3	5	55.6
[l]	33	4.9	17	51.5
[j]	2	.3	1	50.0
[w]	38	5.6	17	44.7
[r]	53	7.8	22	41.5
[v]	18	2.7	7	38.9
[m]	26	3.8	9	34.6
[p]	21	3.1	7	33.3
[n]	57	8.4	19	33.3
[dʒ]	7	1.0	2	28.6
[ʃ]	11	1.6	3	27.3
[f]	21	3.1	5	23.8
[k]	34	5.0	8	23.5
[tʃ]	10	1.5	2	20.0
[s]	33	4.9	6	18.2
[b]	22	3.2	4	18.2
[g]	7	1.0	1	14.3
[t]	67	9.9	9	13.4
[z]	32	4.7	4	12.5
[ʒ]	1	.1	0	0
[ʍ]	2	.3	0	0

Tables 32 and 33 show that ten sounds were produced correctly every time they were spoken by the high intelligibility group, while no sound was always produced correctly by the low intelligibility group. The percentages of errors for each sound excepting the [ʍ] and [h] indicate the consonant sounds were incorrectly produced more often by the low intelligibility laryngectomized group, revealing that for this **group lower** intelligibility is related to the higher percentage of consonant errors produced.

TABLE 31

CONSONANT SOUNDS RANKED ACCORDING TO DIFFICULTY, OCCURRENCE
OF SOUNDS, PERCENTAGE OF OCCURRENCE OF EACH SOUND, NUMBER
OF ERRORS FOR EACH SOUND AND PERCENTAGE OF ERRORS FOR
EACH SOUND FOR THE 750 PB WORDS SPOKEN BY THE
FIFTEEN LARYNGECTOMIZED SPEAKERS

Sounds Ranked in Order of Difficulty	Occurrence of Sounds	Percent of Occurrence of Sounds	Number of Errors for Sounds	Percent of Errors of Sounds
[ʍ]	7	.6	7	100
[j]	3	.3	3	100
[h]	35	3.2	34	97.1
[ð]	12	1.1	6	50.0
[ʒ]	2	.2	1	50.0
[n]	55	5.0	24	43.6
[z]	30	2.7	12	40.0
[θ]	19	1.7	7	36.8
[p]	85	7.7	28	32.9
[g]	51	4.6	16	31.4
[l]	58	5.2	18	31.0
[v]	29	2.6	9	31.0
[m]	48	4.3	14	29.2
[ŋ]	7	.6	2	28.6
[dʒ]	32	2.9	9	28.1
[r]	72	6.5	19	26.4
[f]	66	6.0	16	24.2
[ʃ]	44	4.0	10	22.7
[d]	98	8.8	19	19.4
[t]	81	7.3	14	17.3
[tʃ]	30	2.7	4	13.3
[k]	87	7.8	11	12.6
[b]	60	5.4	7	11.7
[w]	29	2.6	3	10.3
[s]	69	6.2	5	7.2

TABLE 32

CONSONANT SOUNDS RANKED ACCORDING TO DIFFICULTY, OCCURRENCE
OF SOUNDS, PERCENTAGE OF OCCURRENCE OF EACH SOUND, NUMBER
OF ERRORS FOR EACH SOUND AND PERCENTAGE OF ERRORS FOR
EACH SOUND FOR THE 750 PB WORDS SPOKEN BY THE
SEVEN HIGH INTELLIGIBILITY
LARYNGECTOMIZED SPEAKERS

Sounds Ranked in Order of Difficulty	Occurrence of Sounds	Percent of Occurrence of Sounds	Number of Errors for Sounds	Percent of Errors of Sounds
[h]	15	2.9	15	100
[ʍ]	2	.4	2	100
[θ]	8	1.6	2	25.0
[p]	35	6.8	7	20.0
[l]	28	5.4	5	17.9
[ð]	6	1.2	1	16.7
[dʒ]	18	3.5	2	11.1
[v]	18	3.5	2	11.1
[n]	21	4.1	2	9.5
[r]	26	5.0	2	7.7
[f]	30	5.8	2	6.7
[d]	47	9.1	3	6.4
[k]	44	8.5	2	4.5
[m]	28	5.4	1	3.6
[b]	26	5.0	0	0
[g]	24	4.7	0	0
[s]	37	7.2	0	0
[z]	7	1.4	0	0
[ʃ]	20	3.9	0	0
[ʒ]	1	.2	0	0
[tʃ]	12	2.3	0	0
[ŋ]	4	.8	0	0
[j]	0	0	0	0
[w]	15	2.9	0	0

TABLE 33

CONSONANT SOUNDS RANKED ACCORDING TO DIFFICULTY, OCCURRENCE
OF SOUNDS, PERCENTAGE OF OCCURRENCE OF EACH SOUND, NUMBER
OF ERRORS FOR EACH SOUND AND PERCENTAGE OF ERRORS FOR
EACH SOUND FOR THE 750 PB WORDS SPOKEN BY THE
EIGHT LOW INTELLIGIBILITY
LARYNGECTOMIZED SPEAKERS

Sounds Ranked in Order of Difficulty	Occurrence of Sounds	Percent of Occurrence of Sounds	Number of Errors for Sounds	Percent of Errors of Sounds
[ʒ]	1	.2	1	100
[ʍ]	5	.8	5	100
[j]	3	.5	3	100
[h]	20	3.4	19	95.0
[ð]	6	1.0	5	83.3
[ŋ]	3	.5	2	66.7
[m]	20	3.4	13	65.0
[n]	34	5.7	22	64.7
[v]	11	1.9	7	63.6
[g]	27	4.6	16	59.3
[z]	23	3.9	12	52.2
[dʒ]	14	2.4	7	50.0
[θ]	11	1.9	5	45.5
[l]	30	5.1	13	43.3
[p]	50	8.4	21	42.0
[ʃ]	24	4.0	10	41.7
[f]	36	6.1	14	38.9
[r]	46	7.8	17	37.0
[t]	37	6.2	12	32.4
[d]	51	8.6	16	31.4
[tʃ]	18	3.0	4	22.2
[w]	14	2.4	3	21.4
[k]	43	7.3	9	20.9
[b]	34	5.7	7	20.6
[s]	32	5.4	5	15.6

RHYTHM ANALYSIS

Analysis of intelligibility requires a consideration of rhythm as a factor.

Hudgins and Numbers, who investigated the speech intelligibility of 192 deaf children, included a consideration of the rhythm factor:

> Speech rhythm is a specific form of rhythm; it is based upon the syllable rate, the word accent, and the proper grouping of syllables about this accent in the formation of breath groups regulated by the breathing muscles. . . . (27), p. 357.

> Sentences spoken rhythmically correct by deaf pupils have almost a four to one (3.5 to 1) advantage of being understood over those spoken with incorrect rhythm. Slightly less than half (45 per cent) of all sentences spoken by 192 deaf pupils were spoken with normal rhythm, yet these accounted for three-fourths (74 per cent) of all the sentences understood by the auditors. The remaining sentences spoken with abnormal rhythm or with no rhythm (55 per cent) accounted for only 26 per cent of all sentences understood by the auditors. (27), p. 352.

Table 34 indicates results of the rhythm analysis in this study. Eighty-one, or 54 per cent, of the total 150 sentences were spoken with normal rhythm. Abnormal rhythm was present in 55, or 37 per cent, of the total number of sentences, and sentences spoken non-rhythmically accounted for 14, or 9 per cent, of the total number of sentences. Sixty-eight per cent of the normal rhythm sentences were understood. Conversely, only 21 per cent of the abnormal sentences were understood, and 11 per cent of non-rhythmical sentences were understood. These values show marked

TABLE 34

NUMBER AND PERCENT OF SENTENCES FOUND TO BE NORMAL IN RHYTHM,
ABNORMAL IN RHYTHM, OR NON-RHYTHMICAL, WITH PERCENT OF
TOTAL SENTENCES UNDERSTOOD AND PERCENT OF
UNDERSTOOD SENTENCES IN EACH CATEGORY

Rhythm Categories	Number of Sentences Spoken	Percent of Total Number of Sentences	Percent of Total Sentences Understood	Percent of Total Understood Sentences in Each Category
Normal	81	54	68	89
Abnormal	55	37	21	40
Non-rhythmical	14	9	11	82
Total	150	100	100	

similarity to the values that Hudgins and Numbers report, and indicate
the possibilities of rhythm as a predictor of intelligibility for the speech
of the laryngectomized. In considering the per cent of total understood
sentences in each category, 89 per cent of the normal rhythm sentences
and 82 per cent of the non-rhythmical sentences were understood and 40
per cent of the abnormal sentences were understood. Indications here
are that not all sentences spoken with correct rhythm are understood, or
that all sentences spoken with abnormal rhythm are not understood. It
appears that other variables may be operating in this situation.

Figure 39 illustrates the number of sentences spoken with normal
rhythm for the laryngectomized individuals. The mean of 5.40 sentences
is based on a total of ten sentences spoken by each speaker. Here again
we see evidence of a group of laryngectomized speakers above and below
the mean.

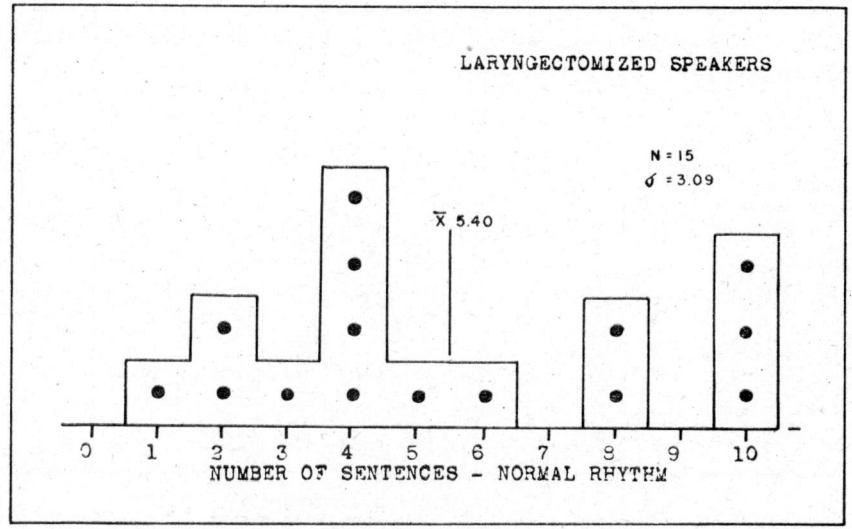

FIG. 39. Distribution of number of sentences having normal rhythm for the
laryngectomized individuals, showing x̄, N, and σ.

HIGH AND LOW INTELLIGIBILITY GROUPS

COMPARISONS OF THE LARYNGECTOMIZED SPEAKERS AND THE NORMAL
SPEAKERS ON VARIABLES WITH PREDICTIVE VALUE FOR INTELLIGIBILITY

The analysis of the data has substantiated the hypothesis that the quantitative intelligibility indexes used in this investigation would differentiate between the laryngectomized speakers. A second hypothesis is that laryngectomized speakers who are most intelligible would approximate more closely the speech coordinations of the normal speakers. To examine this hypothesis comparisons were made between the normal group and the $+\bar{z}$ and the $-\bar{z}$ groups of laryngectomized speakers. The speech coordinations for the sixty-syllable paragraph serves as a basis of

TABLE 35

MEANS, VARIANCES, DIFFERENCES BETWEEN MEANS, t AND F VALUES; TIME, NUMBER
OF PHRASES, TIME PER PHRASE, NUMBER OF SYLLABLES PER PHRASE; AND
ABDOMINAL, CHEST AND COMBINED AMPLITUDE IN MILLIMETERS FOR
THE NORMAL SPEAKERS AND FOR THE LARYNGECTOMIZED SPEAKERS
WITH +z AND -z̄ INTELLIGIBILITY SCORES

Variables	Normal Group			$+\bar{z}$ Group			$-\bar{z}$ Group		
	$\bar{X}$	σ^2	σ	$\bar{X}$	σ^2	σ	$\bar{X}$	σ^2	σ
Time	19.14	7.42	2.72	24.37	16.88	4.11	60.81	999.06	31.61
Number of phrases	5.20	2.60	1.61	15.43	46.95	6.85	37.88	214.41	14.64
Time per phrase	3.92	1.08	1.03	1.84	.56	.75	1.62	.44	.67
Number of syllables per phrase	12.52	12.7	3.57	4.65	4.27	2.07	1.78	.34	.59
Abdominal amplitude, millimeters	9.93	13.5	3.67	8.67	15.68	3.96	10.21	11.39	3.38
Chest amplitude, millimeters	13.11	24.3	4.93	11.09	26.99	5.20	11.54	18.80	4.34
Combined amplitude, millimeters	11.52	11.0	3.32	9.88	10.47	3.24	10.88	7.51	2.74

Table value of t recalculated according to
Cochran and Cox formula employed when comparing groups
of different N's when variances differ significantly.

Found in Edwards, Experimental Design in
Psychological Research, Formula 55, p. 168.

comparison for this analysis. The data for this speech sample reveal significant differences between the laryngectomized speakers as a group and the normal speakers for the variables:

1. total time in speaking the sixty-syllable paragraph,
2. number of phrases employed in speaking the sixty-syllable paragraph.

A question arising from the analysis is whether the high intelligibility group would more closely approach the coordinations of the normal speakers than the low intelligibility group. The data for this question are summarized in Table 35.

FOR THE TIME VARIABLE

The normal group has a mean of 19.14 seconds for speaking the sixty-syllable paragraph, while the high has a mean of 24.37 seconds. This difference of 5.23 seconds is significant at the .01 level of confidence. When

TABLE 35--Continued

Comparisons $+\bar{z}$ - Normal				Comparisons $-\bar{z}$ - Normal				Comparisons $(-\bar{z})$ - $(+\bar{z})$				
$\bar{X}_{+z}\bar{X}_n$	t	Cal.t / t.01	F	$\bar{X}_{-z}\bar{X}_n$	t	Cal.t / t.01	F	$\bar{X}_{-z}\bar{X}_{+z}$	t	Cal. t / t.01	t.05	F
5.23	3.56**		2.27	41.67	3.72**	3.50	134.60**	36.44	3.23*	3.50	2.37	59.19**
10.23	3.90**	3.69	18.06	32.68	6.29**	3.50	82.47**	22.45	3.70**			4.57
-2.08	4.74**		1.93	-2.30	9.48**		2.42	- .22	.60			1.25
-7.87	5.39*		2.97	-10.74	11.38**	3.00	36.87**	-2.87	3.55*	3.69		12.39**
-1.26	.73		1.16	.28	.22		1.15	1.54	.81			1.38
-2.02	.88		1.11	-1.57	.96		1.29	.45	.18			1.44
-1.64	1.29		1.05	- .64	.62		1.47	1.00	.65			1.39

** = t significant at .01 level (3.012)   ** = F significant at
 * = t significant at .05 level (2.160)   .02 level (8.26)

xx = .01 level   Indicates significance
 x = .05 level   of t when F is
                 significant

the lows are compared to the normals on this variable, the mean time for the lows is 60.81 seconds. This difference between the means of the lows and the normals is 41.67, which is significant at the .01 level of confidence. The F of 134.60 is highly significant. When the t is calculated in view of the significant F the t remains significant at the .01 level of confidence. In this situation for time both the high and the low differ significantly from the normal. However, a consideration of the differences between the means for these groups indicates marked differences. The highs and normals were separated for approximately a five-second interval, while the lows spoke the sixty-syllable paragraph in a period approximately forty-two seconds greater than the normals. While differences exist between the highs and the normals, the greater differences existing between lows and the normals and the lows and the highs are not only statistically significant, but also become meaningful in a communicative sense.

For the Number of Phrases Variable

The normal group spoke the sixty-syllable paragraph in 5.20 phrases; the high group in 15.43 phrases; and the low group in 37.8 phrases. The data reveal that the normals differ significantly from both the high and the low groups. Nevertheless, when the same comparison is made for phrases that is made for time in respect to the differences between the means of the normal and the high, and the normal and the low, it is revealed that the lows speak the paragraph using approximately three times the number of phrases as do the high when compared to the normals. The difference between the mean and the normal is approximately ten phrases, while the difference beween the mean of the low and the normal is approximately thirty-three phrases. The amplitude measurements for the abdominal, chest and combined do not reveal significant difference between the groups.

Figures 40 and 41 indicate clearly the similarity beween the laryngectomized speakers with high intelligibility and the normal group, and the variability between the laryngectomized speakers with low intelligibility and the normal group for the predictors, time and phrases.

To summarize, the hypothesis which states that the better laryngectomized speakers will approach the normal speech coordinations more closely than the poorer laryngectomized has been substantiated. Although the statistical data reveal that the laryngectomized who are high in intelligibility differ significantly from the normal group on the variables measured, they also differ significantly from the laryngectomized speakers who are judged to be low in intelligibility. In addition, when considered from the standpoint of meaningful communicative situations, the large differences between the laryngectomized who are low in intelligibility and the normals, and the smaller differences between the laryngectomized who are high in intelligibility and the normals, the contrast becomes an operational one.

EVALUATION OF ARTICULATORY DIFFERENCES BETWEEN HIGH AND LOW INTELLIGIBILITY GROUPS

Table 36 presents the mean, variance, standard deviation, difference between the means, t and F values for the consonant errors for the sentence material for seven high and eight low intelligibility groups of

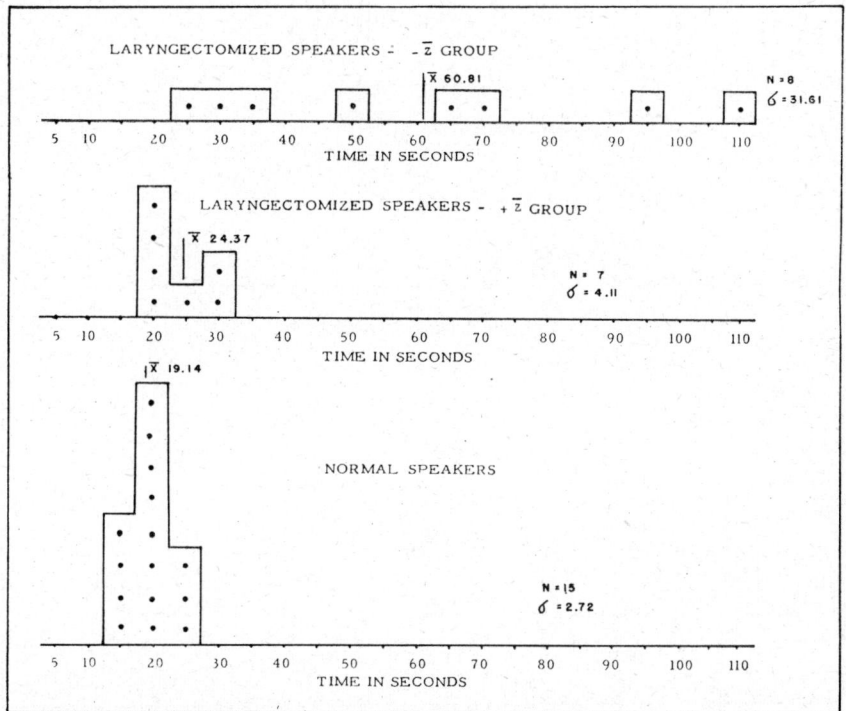

FIG. 40. Distribution per total time in seconds for the sixty-syllable paragraph for the laryngectomized subjects divided into two groups, (1) those higher than the mean on the combined intelligibility score ($+\bar{z}$ group) and (2) those lower than the mean on the combined intelligibility score ($-\bar{z}$ group) compared with the normal speakers, indicating $\bar{x}$, N, and σ for the three groups.

laryngectomized speakers. The high intelligibility group has a mean of 15.29 consonant errors and the low intelligibility group has a mean of 36.25 consonant errors. The difference between the means is 20.96. The t value of 4.75 is significant beyond the .01 level.

Table 37 presents the mean, variance, standard deviation, difference between the means, t and F values for the vowel error categories for the sentence material for seven high and eight low intelligibility groups of laryngectomized speakers. The mean of vowel errors for the low intel-

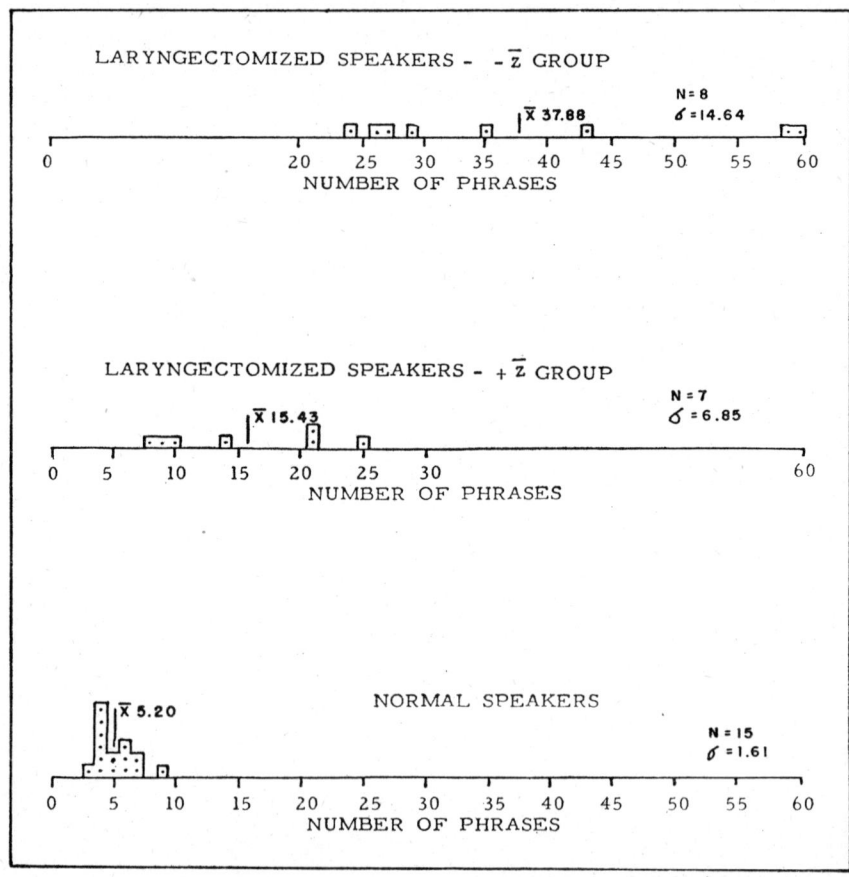

FIG. 41. Distribution of the number of phrases for the sixty-syllable paragraph for the laryngectomized subjects divided into two groups (1) those higher than the mean on the combined intelligibility scores (+z̄ group) and (2) those lower than the mean on the combined intelligibility scores (−z̄ group), compared with the normal speakers, indicating x̄, N, and σ for the three groups.

ligibility group is 10.50. The difference between the means is 8.93. The t value of 5.38 is significant beyond the .01 level.

Table 38 presents the mean, variance, standard deviation, difference between the means, t and F values for the consonant error categories for the PB materials for the seven high and eight low intelligibility groups of laryngectomized speakers. The high intelligibility group has a mean of 9.57 consonant errors and the low intelligibility group has a mean of 39.75. The difference between the means is 30.18. The t value of 11.28 indicates a significance beyond the .01 level.

Table 39 presents the mean, variance, standard deviation, difference between the means, t and F values for the vowel error categories for the PB material for seven high and eight low intelligibility groups of laryngectomized speakers. The mean of vowel errors for the high intelligibility group is 3.86 and the mean of vowel errors for the low intelligibility group is 15.00. The difference between the means is 11.14. The t

TABLE 36

MEANS, VARIANCES, STANDARD DEVIATIONS, DIFFERENCE BETWEEN THE
MEANS, t AND F VALUES FOR THE CONSONANT ERRORS ON
SENTENCES FOR SEVEN HIGH AND EIGHT LOW
INTELLIGIBILITY GROUPS OF
LARYNGECTOMIZED
SPEAKERS

Group	$\overline{X}$	σ^2	σ	$\overline{X}_{+z}-\overline{X}_{-z}$	t	F
Total group N = 15	26.47	184.70	13.59			
High group N_{+z} = 7	15.29	65.94	8.12			
				20.96	4.75**	1.19
Low group $-z$ N = 8	36.25	78.52	8.86			

$$df = N_1 + N_2 - 2 \qquad\qquad df = 7 \text{ and } 6$$

df = 13   F.02 = 8.26
t.01 = 3.012   F.05 = 6.74
t.05 = 2.160   (Interpolated)
          F.10 = 4.21

** = .01
* = .05   ** = .02
           * = .05

value indicates a significant difference between the means beyond the .01 level but the F value of 9.52 is also significant, necessitating a recalculation of the t. The recalculated t value is 3.79 and remains significant beyond the .05 level.

Table 40 presents the number of possible errors and the number and corresponding percentages of correct sounds in the various categories for the sentences for the seven high and eight low intelligibility laryngectomized speakers. The table reveals that the high intelligibility laryngectomized speakers produced correctly at least 90 per cent of all sounds in both consonant and vowel categories. The table also reveals a closer approximation between both groups for vowel production than for consonant production. The difference between the high and low groups contrasts for the compound, releasing and arresting consonants. Figures 42 through 48 illustrate these relationships for the sentence material.

TABLE 37

MEANS, VARIANCES, STANDARD DEVIATIONS, DIFFERENCE BETWEEN THE MEANS, t AND F VALUES FOR THE VOWEL ERRORS ON SENTENCES FOR SEVEN HIGH AND EIGHT LOW INTELLIGIBILITY GROUPS OF LARYNGECTOMIZED SPEAKERS

Group	$\overline{X}$	σ^2	σ	$\overline{X}_{+\overline{z}}-\overline{X}_{-\overline{z}}$	t	F
Total group N = 15	6.33	30.81	5.55			
High group +$\overline{z}$ N = 7	1.57	3.95	1.99			
				8.93	5.38**	3.98
Low group -$\overline{z}$ N = 8	10.50	15.72	3.96			

$$df = N_1 + N_2 - 2 \qquad\qquad df = 7 \text{ and } 6$$

$$df = 13 \qquad\qquad F.02 = 8.26$$
$$t_{01} = 3.012 \qquad\qquad F.05 = 6.74$$
$$t_{.05} = 2.160 \qquad\qquad\qquad (\text{Interpolated})$$
$$F.10 = 4.21$$

$$** = .01 \qquad\qquad\qquad ** = .02$$
$$* = .05 \qquad\qquad\qquad * = .05$$

Table 41 shows the number of possible errors, the number and percentages of correct sounds in the various categories in the PB monosyllabic words for the seven high and eight low intelligibility laryngectomized speakers. This table also reveals that the high intelligibility laryngectomized speakers produced correctly at least 90 per cent of all sounds in both consonant and vowel categories for the PB materials. Furthermore, the production of vowels was equally consistent for both groups. In the consonant categories, however, a difference appears in the production of the surd-sonant, substitution and compound consonant categories. The releasing and arresting consonants which reveal differences in Table 40 were produced equally well by both groups for the PB materials. Figures 49 through 55 also illustrate these relationships.

TABLE 38

MEANS, VARIANCES, STANDARD DEVIATIONS, DIFFERENCE BETWEEN THE
MEANS,   t   AND   F   VALUES FOR THE CONSONANT ERRORS
ON PB WORDS FOR SEVEN HIGH AND EIGHT LOW
INTELLIGIBILITY GROUPS OF
LARYNGECTOMIZED
SPEAKERS

Group	$\overline{X}$	σ^2	σ	$\overline{X}_{+\overline{z}}-\overline{X}_{-\overline{z}}$	t	F
Total group N = 15	25.67	267.67	16.36			
High group +z̄ N = 7	9.57	11.29	3.36			
				30.18	11.28[**]	3.54
Low group -z̄ N = 8	39.75	39.93	6.32			

$$df = N_1 + N_2 - 2 \qquad\qquad df = 7 \text{ and } 6$$

df = 13 $F_{.02}$ = 8.26
$t_{.01}$ = 3.012 $F_{.05}$ = 6.74
$t_{.05}$ = 2.160   (Interpolated)
                                 $F_{.10}$ = 4.21
** = .01
 * = .05   ** = .02
                                  * = .05

Table 42 presents the ranking of the vowel and consonant categories according to the percentages of sounds incorrectly produced for the sentences for the high and low intelligibility groups. The greatest differences between the two groups appear in the arresting, compound and releasing consonants. For the high intelligibility group the arresting consonants rank eighth, the compound consonants tenth, and the releasing consonants eleventh. Nevertheless, the production of incorrect sounds was less than 9 per cent in all these categories. For the low intelligibility group the releasing, compound and arresting consonants are ranked ninth, tenth and eleventh, respectively, but the highest percent-

TABLE 39

MEANS, VARIANCES, STANDARD DEVIATIONS, DIFFERENCE BETWEEN THE
MEANS, t AND F VALUES FOR THE VOWEL ERRORS ON
PB WORDS FOR SEVEN HIGH AND EIGHT LOW
INTELLIGIBILITY GROUPS OF
LARYNGECTOMIZED
SPEAKERS

Group	$\overline{X}$	σ^2	σ	$\overline{X}_{-\bar{z}} - \overline{X}_{+\bar{z}}$	t	F
Total group N = 15	9.80	66.74	8.17			
High group +$\bar{z}$ N = 7	3.86	6.48	2.54			
				11.14	3.79^x	9.52^{**}
Low group -$\bar{z}$ N = 8	15.00	61.71	7.86			

df = N_1 + N_2 - 2   df = 7 and 6

df = 13
t.01 = 3.012
t.05 = 2.160

F.02 = 8.26
F.05 = 6.74
                    (Interpolated)
F.10 = 4.21

** = .01
* = .05

** = .02
* = .05

x = .05 level   Indicates significance
of t when F is
significant.

age of incorrect production is 29.5 for the arresting consonants. Figure 56 is a bar graph which reveals the relationships presented in Table 42.

Table 43 presents the mean, variance, standard deviation, difference between the means, t and F values and corrected t's when the F value is significant for consonant error categories for the sentence material for seven high and eight low intelligibility groups of laryngectomized speakers.

In the arresting and releasing consonants the F values are significant. Therefore, the t values have to be corrected. When the t values are corrected, the arresting consonant still remains significant beyond the .01 level, while the releasing consonant remains significant beyond the .05 level. The t value for the compound consonant is not significant. The t value for surd-sonant proves to be significant beyond the .01 level. The t values for the vowel errors indicate that for the neutralization and omission categories the difference between the means is significant beyond · .01 level, while the difference between the means for the constructive

TABLE 40

THE NUMBER OF POSSIBLE ERRORS AND THE NUMBER AND CORRESPONDING PERCENTAGES OF CORRECT SOUNDS IN THE VARIOUS CATEGORIES FOR THE SENTENCES FOR SEVEN HIGH AND EIGHT LOW INTELLIGIBILITY LARYNGECTOMIZED SPEAKERS

	Categories	Number of Possible Errors		Number of Correct Sounds		Percent of Correct Sounds	
		High	Low	High	Low	High	Low
Consonants	Surd-sonant	357	414	350	381	98.2	92.0
	Substitution	706	790	664	719	94.1	91.0
	Compound consonants	123	117	113	91	91.9	77.8
	Releasing consonants	310	439	285	368	91.9	83.9
	Arresting consonants	233	227	226	160	96.9	70.5
	Constructive compound	706	790	690	768	97.7	97.2
Vowels	Substitution	487	576	484	559	99.3	97.0
	Diphthongization	387	472	385	470	99.4	99.7
	Neutralization	487	576	487	569	100	98.7
	Omission	487	576	487	545	100	94.6
	Constructive release	487	576	481	549	98.7	95.4

release is significant beyond the .05 level. Inspection of the data reveals that six of the eleven categories show significant differences between the means beyond either the .01 or .05 level.

Table 44 indicates the ranking of the consonant and vowel categories according to the percentages of sounds incorrectly produced for the phonetically balanced monosyllabic words for the high and low intelligibility groups of laryngectomized speakers. Table 42 indicates that for the sentence material the releasing, compound and arresting consonants for the low intelligibility group were incorrectly produced 19.9, 22.2 and 29.5 per cent respectively. Table 44 shows a shift in this relationship for both the releasing and arresting consonants, while the compound consonants retain the same rank. While for the sentences the releasing consonants were incorrectly produced 19.9 per cent and are ranked ninth. In the PB material the categories shift from ninth position to third

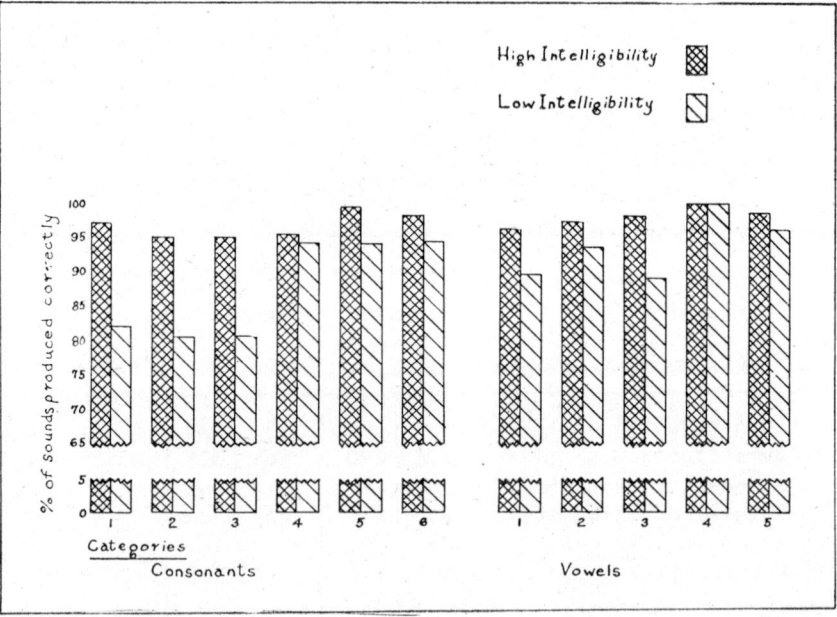

Fig. 42. Percentages of sounds produced correctly in the various consonant and vowel error categories for the seven high and eight low intelligibility laryngectomized speakers for the sentences.

Consonant error categories: 1) surd-sonant, 2) substitution, 3) compound consonant, 4) releasing consonant, 5) arresting consonant, 6) constructive compound.

Vowel error categories: 1) substitution, 2) diphthongization, 3) neutralization, 4) omission, 5) constructive release.

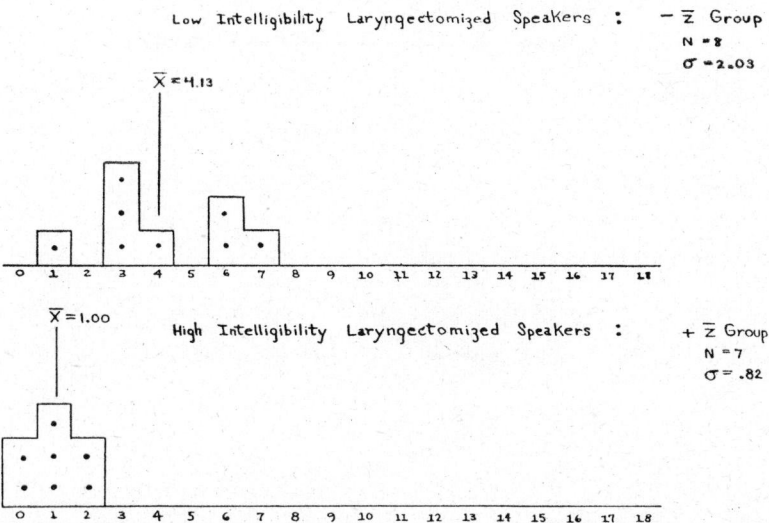

FIG. 43. Distribution of the number of errors in the surd-sonant consonant error category for each of the seven high and eight low intelligibility laryngectomized speakers for the sentences, showing x̄, N and σ for each group.

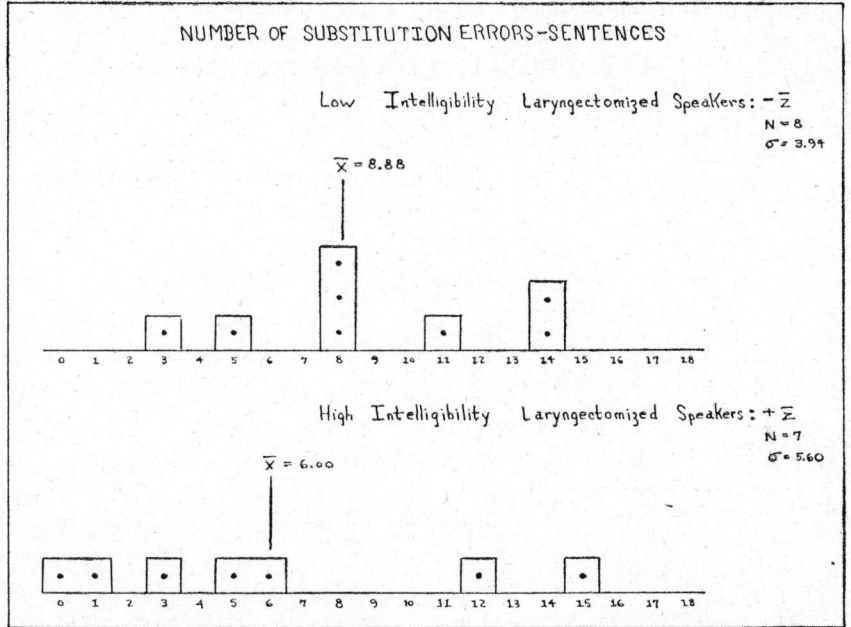

FIG. 44. Distribution of the number of errors in the substitution consonant error category for each of the seven high and eight low intelligibility laryngectomized speakers for the sentences, showing x̄, N and σ for each group.

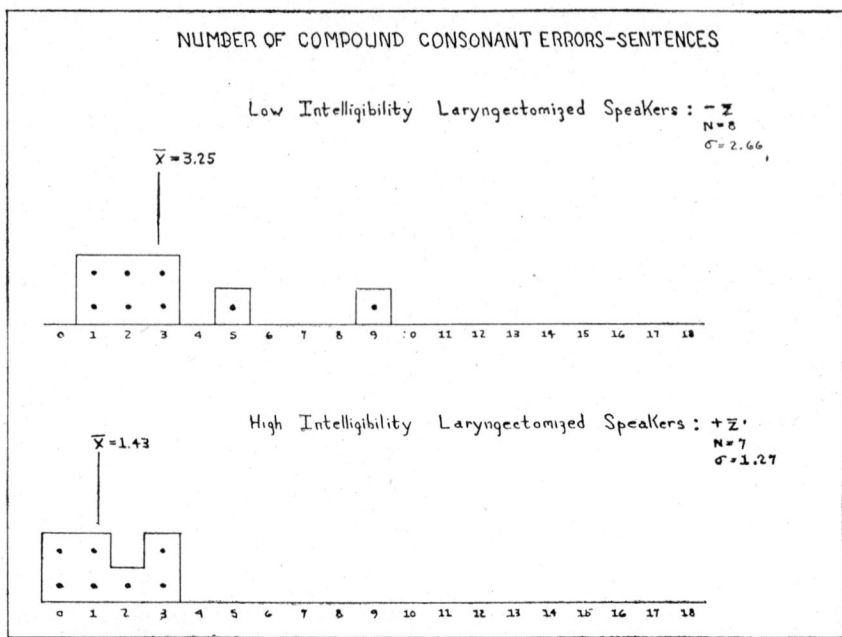

FIG. 45. Distribution of the number of errors in the compound consonant error category for each of the seven high and eight low intelligibility laryngectomized speakers for the sentences, showing x̄, N and σ for each group.

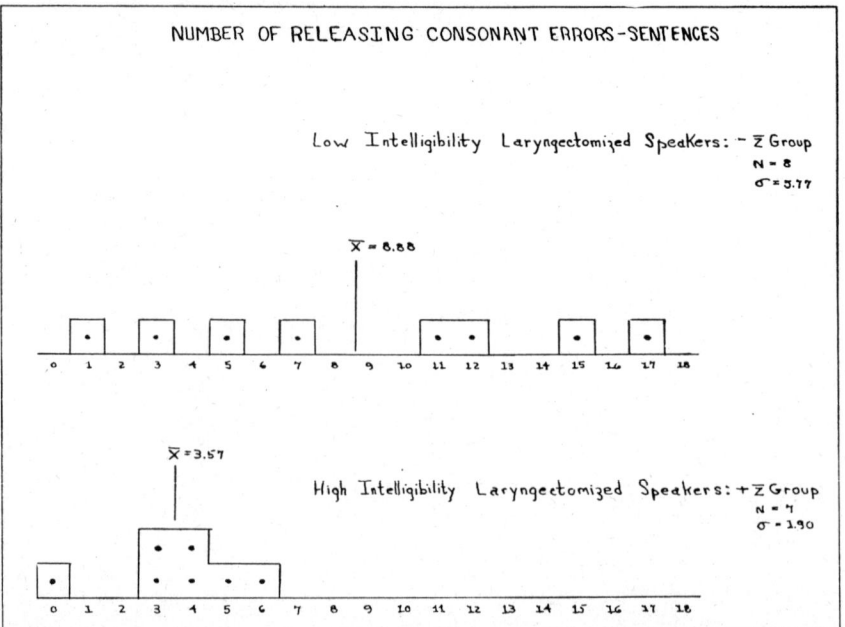

FIG. 46. Distribution of the number of errors in the releasing consonant error category for each of the seven high and eight low intelligibility laryngectomized speakers for the sentences, showing x̄, N and σ for each group.

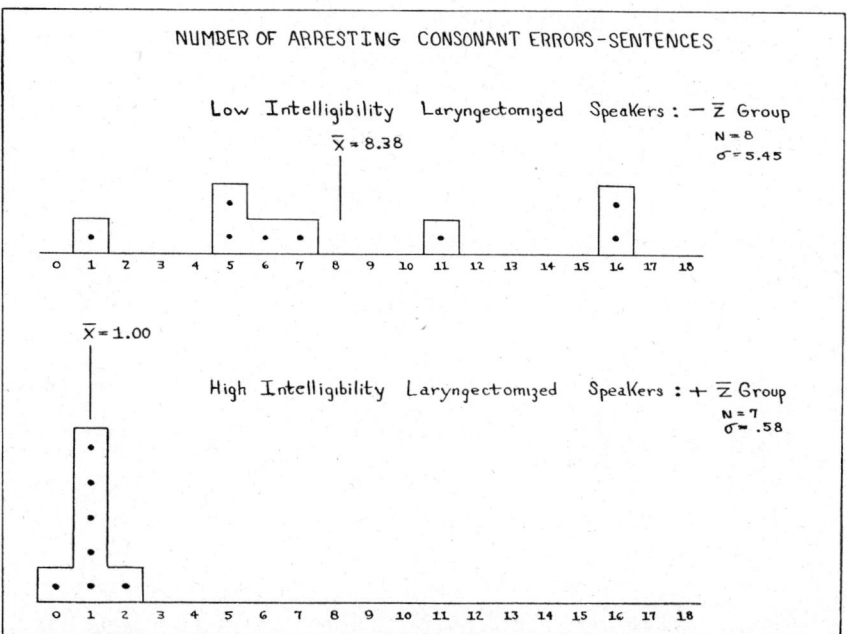

Fig. 47. Distribution of the number of errors in the arresting consonant error category for each of the seven high and eight low intelligibility laryngectomized speakers for the sentences, showing $\bar{x}$, N and σ for each group.

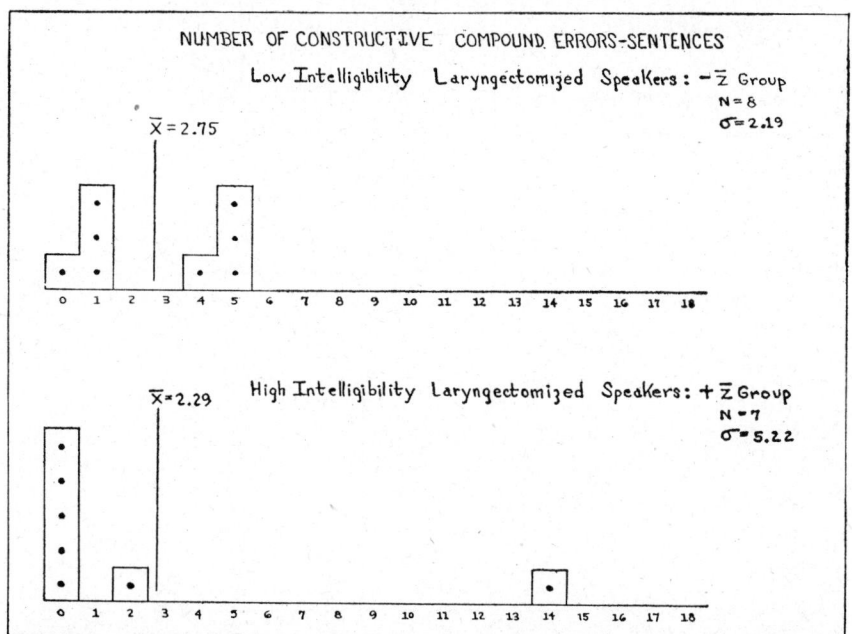

Fig. 48. Distribution of the number of errors in the constructive compound error category for each of the seven high and eight low intelligibility laryngectomized speakers for the sentences, showing $\bar{x}$, N and σ for each group.

TABLE 41

THE NUMBER OF POSSIBLE ERRORS AND NUMBER AND PERCENTAGES
OF CORRECT SOUNDS IN THE VARIOUS CATEGORIES IN THE
PHONETICALLY BALANCED MONOSYLLABIC WORDS FOR
SEVEN HIGH AND EIGHT LOW INTELLIGIBILITY
LARYNGECTOMIZED SPEAKERS

	Categories	Number of Possible Errors		Number of Times Produced Correctly		Percent of Times Produced Correctly	
		High	Low	High	Low	High	Low
Consonants	Surd-sonant	377	418	366	343	97.1	82.1
	Substitution	636	734	604	591	95.0	80.5
	Compound consonants	120	141	114	114	95.0	80.9
	Releasing consonants	259	291	248	275	95.4	94.5
	Arresting consonants	236	290	235	273	99.5	94.1
	Constructive compound	636	734	630	694	98.2	94.6
Vowels	Substitution	343	402	330	360	96.2	89.9
	Diphthongization	238	289	232	271	97.4	93.7
	Neutralization	343	402	337	358	98.2	89.0
	Omission	343	402	343	402	100	100
	Constructive release	343	402	339	386	98.8	96.0

TABLE 42

RANKING OF THE VOWEL AND CONSONANT CATEGORIES ACCORDING TO THE
PERCENTAGES OF SOUNDS INCORRECTLY PRODUCED FOR THE SENTENCES
FOR THE SEVEN HIGH AND EIGHT LOW INTELLIGIBILITY
LARYNGECTOMIZED SPEAKERS

High Intelligibility Group		Low Intelligibility Group		Total Group	
Error Categories	Percent Errors	Error Categories	Percent Errors	Error Categories	Percent Errors
Omission	0	Diphthongization	.3	Diphthongization	.4
Neutralization	0	Neutralization	1.3	Neutralization	.8
Diphthongization	.6	Constructive compound	2.8	Vowel substitution	1.9
Vowel substitution	.7	Vowel substitution	3.0	Omission	2.4
Constructive release	1.3	Constructive release	4.6	Constructive compound	2.5
Surd-sonant	2.0	Omission	5.4	Constructive release	3.1
Constructive compound	2.3	Surd-sonant	8.0	Surd-sonant	5.2
Arresting consonants	3.1	Consonant substitution	9.0	Consonant substitution	7.6
Consonant substitution	5.9	Releasing consonants	19.9	Releasing consonants	12.8
Compound consonants	8.1	Compound consonants	22.2	Compound consonants	15.0
Releasing consonants	8.1	Arresting consonants	29.5	Arresting consonants	16.1

TABLE 43

MEANS, VARIANCES STANDARD DEVIATIONS, DIFFERENCES BETWEEN THE MEANS, t AND F VALUES AND CORRECTED t WHEN THE F VALUE IS SIGNIFICANT FOR THE CONSONANT AND VOWEL ERROR CATEGORIES FOR SENTENCES FOR THE SEVEN HIGH AND EIGHT LOW INTELLIGIBILITY GROUPS OF LARYNGECTOMIZED SPEAKERS

Variables	High +z̄ Group			Low -z̄ Group			X̄+z̄-X̄-z	t	Cal.t .05	F
	X̄	σ²	σ	X̄	σ²	σ				
Total consonants	15.29	65.94	8.12	36.25	78.52	8.86	20.96	4.75**		1.19
Total vowels	1.57	3.95	1.99	10.50	15.71	3.96	8.92	5.38**		3.98
Consonants — Surd-sonant	1.00	.67	.82	4.13	4.13	2.03	3.12	3.80**		6.19
Substitution	6.00	31.35	5.60	8.88	15.56	3.94	2.87	1.16		2.01
Compound consonants	1.43	1.62	1.27	3.25	7.07	2.66	1.82	1.65		4.37
Releasing consonants	3.57	3.62	1.90	8.88	33.28	5.77	5.30	2.45x	2.37	9.19**
Arresting consonants	1.00	.33	.58	8.38	29.71	5.45	7.37	3.80x	2.37	89.07**
Constructive compound	2.29	27.25	5.22	2.75	4.79	2.19	.46	.23		5.69
Vowels — Substitution	.43	.62	.79	2.13	4.41	2.10	1.70	2.12	2.38	7.12*
Diphthongization	.29	.24	.49	.25	.21	.46	-.04	-.15		1.11
Neutralization	0.00	0.00	0.00	.88	.41	.64	.88	3.59**		0.00
Omission	0.00	0.00	0.00	3.88	10.41	3.23	3.88	3.16**		0.00
Constructive release	.86	1.48	1.22	3.38	5.98	2.45	2.52	2.46*		4.05

$$df = N_1 + N_2 - 2$$
$$df = 13$$
$$t_{.01} = 3.012$$
$$t_{.05} = 2.160$$

$$df = 7 \text{ and } 6$$
$$F_{.02} = 8.26$$
$$F_{.05} = 6.74 \quad \text{(Interpolated)}$$
$$F_{.10} = 4.21$$

** = .01
* = .05
xx = .01 level - Indicates
x = .05 level significance of t when F is significant

** = .02
* = .05

TABLE 44

RANKING OF THE CONSONANT AND VOWEL CATEGORIES ACCORDING TO THE PERCENTAGES OF SOUNDS INCORRECTLY PRODUCED FOR THE 750 PHONETICALLY BALANCED MONOSYLLABIC WORDS FOR THE SEVEN HIGH AND EIGHT LOW INTELLIGIBILITY LARYNGECTOMIZED SPEAKERS

High Intelligibility Group		Low Intelligibility Group		Total Group	
Error Categories	Percent of Errors	Error Categories	Percent of Errors	Error Categories	Percent of Errors
Omission	0	Omission	0	Omission	0
Arresting consonants	.5	Constructive release	4.0	Constructive release	2.7
Constructive release	1.2	Constructive compound	5.4	Constructive compound	3.4
Neutralization	1.8	Releasing consonants	5.5	Arresting consonants	3.4
Constructive compound	1.8	Arresting consonants	5.9	Diphthongization	4.6
Diphthongization	2.6	Diphthongization	6.3	Releasing consonants	4.9
Surd-sonant	2.9	Vowel substitution	10.1	Neutralization	6.5
Vowel substitution	3.8	Neutralization	11.0	Vowel substitution	7.4
Releasing consonants	4.6	Surd-sonant	17.9	Surd-sonant	10.8
Consonant substitution	5.0	Compound consonants	19.1	Compound consonants	12.6
Compound consonants	5.0	Consonant substitution	19.5	Consonant substitution	12.8

position with incorrect production 5.5 per cent. The compound consonants are ranked tenth for both materials but for the sentence material they were produced 19.1 per cent incorrectly. The arresting consonants in the sentences are ranked eleventh and were produced 29.5 per cent incorrectly. In the PB material the arresting consonants are ranked fifth and were produced incorrectly 5.9 per cent. Figure 57 indicates these relationships.

Table 45 shows the mean, variance, standard deviation, difference between the means, t and F values and corrected t's when the F value is significant for consonant error categories for the PB material for seven high and eight low intelligibility groups of laryngectomized speakers. In the surd-sonant, compound consonant and arresting consonant categories the F values are significant beyond the .02 level and consequently necessitated correcting the t values. When the t values are corrected the

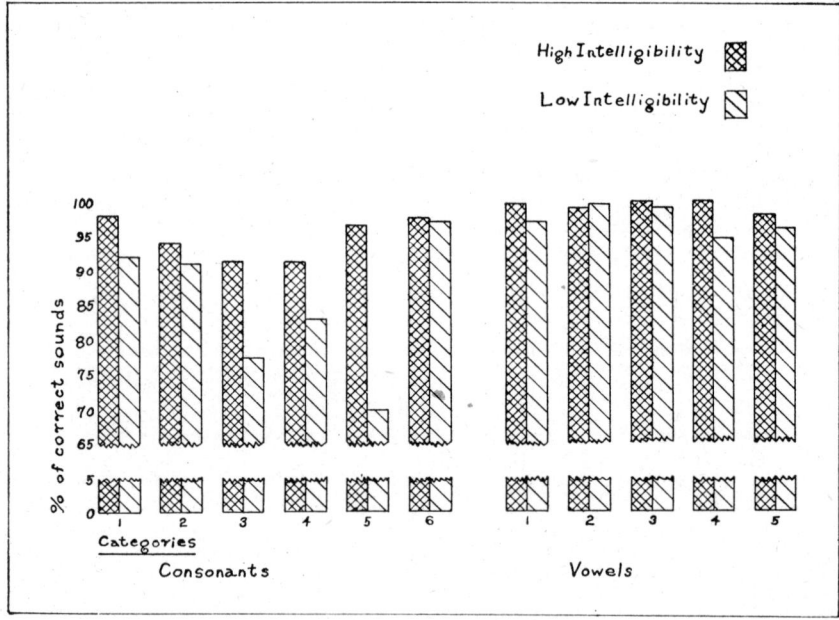

Fig. 49. Percentages of sounds produced correctly in the various consonant and vowel error categories for the seven high and eight low intelligibility laryngectomized speakers for the PB words.

Consonant error categories: 1) surd-sonant, 2) substitution, 3) compound consonant, 4) releasing consonant, 5) arresting consonant, 6) constructive compound.

Vowel error categories: 1) substitution, 2) diphthongization, 3) neutralization, 4) omission, 5) constructive release.

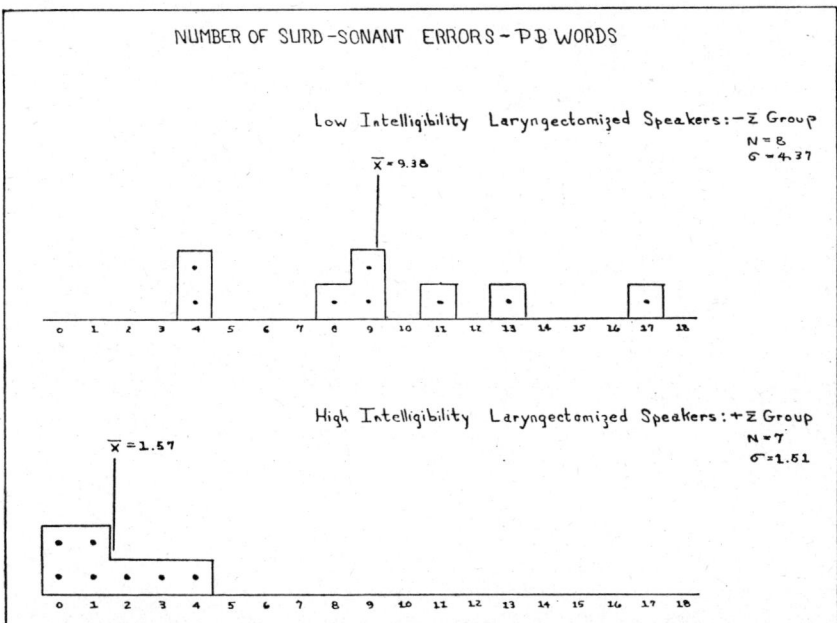

FIG. 50. Distribution of the number of errors in the surd-sonant consonant error category for each of the seven high and eight low intelligibility laryngectomized speakers for the PB words, showing x̄, N and σ for each group.

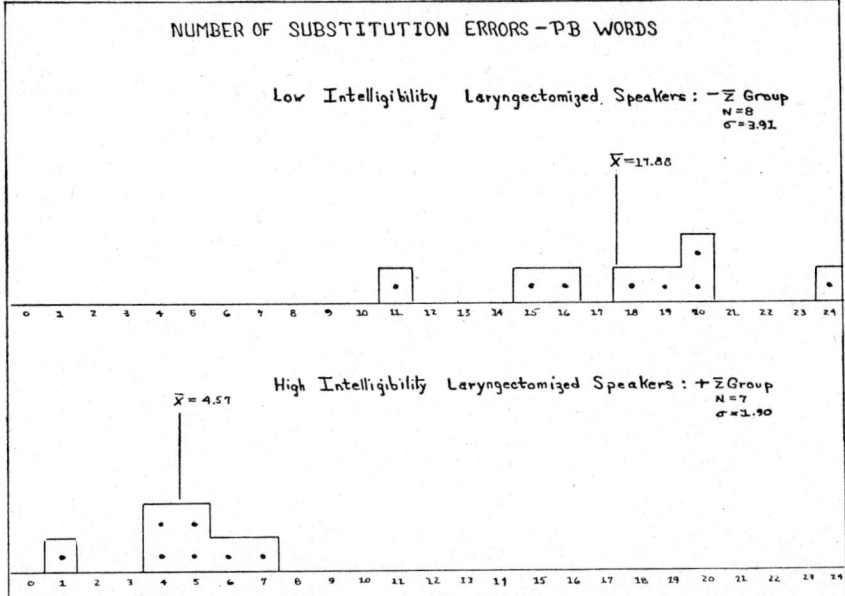

FIG. 51. Distribution of the number of errors in the substitution consonant error category for each of the seven high and eight low intelligibility laryngectomized speakers for the PB words, showing x̄, N and σ for each group.

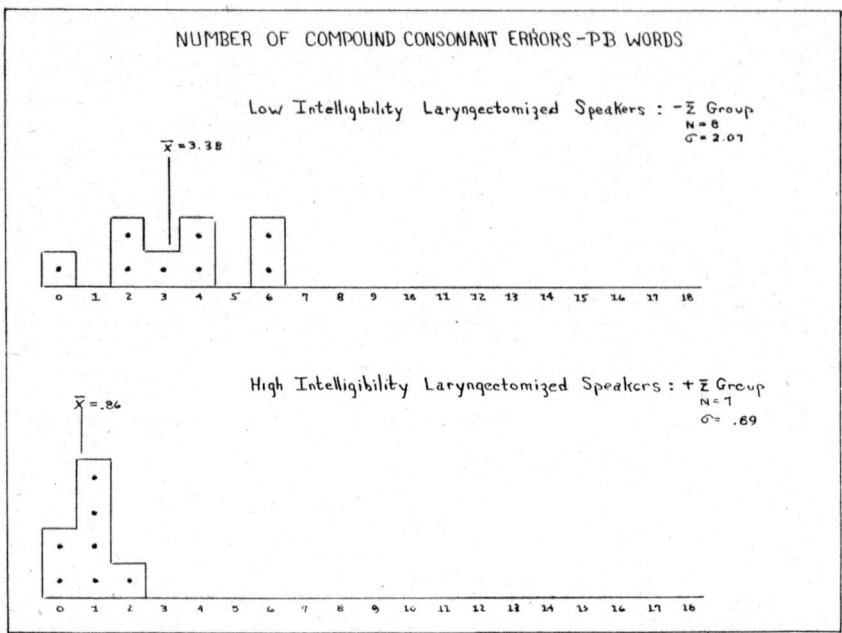

FIG. 52. Distribution of the number of errors in the compound consonant error category for each of the seven high and eight low intelligibility laryngectomized speakers for the PB words, showing x̄, N and σ for each group.

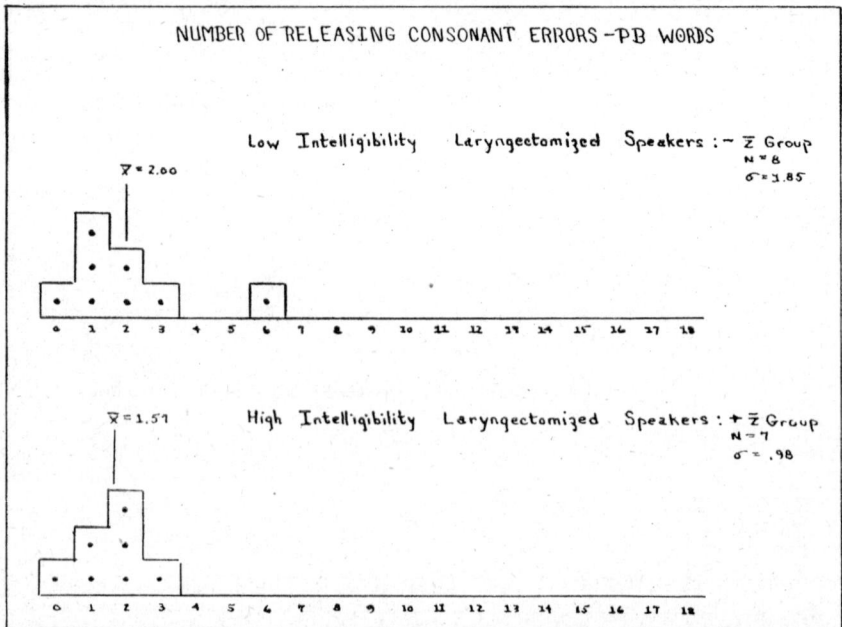

FIG. 53. Distribution of the number of errors in the releasing consonant error category for each of the seven high and eight low intelligibility laryngectomized speakers for the PB words, showing x̄, N and σ for each group.

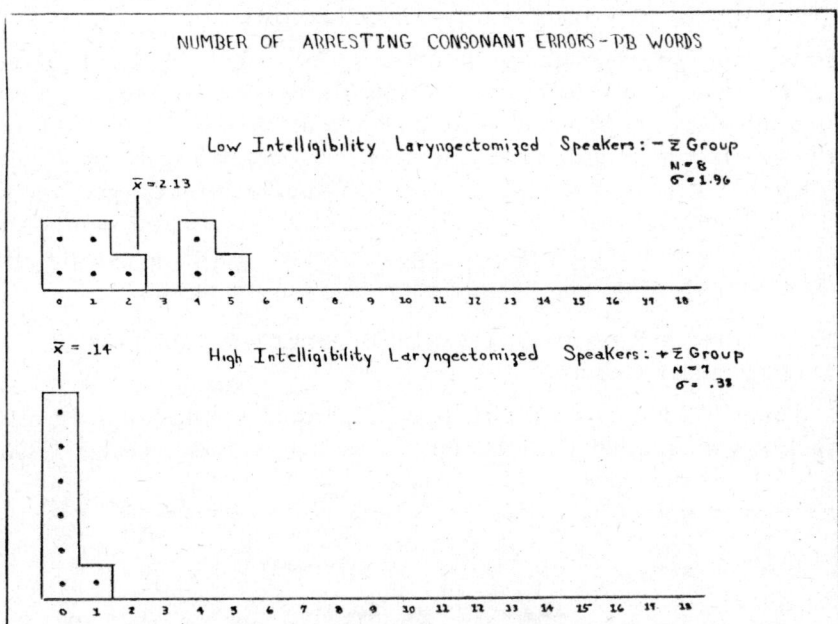

FIG. 54. Distribution of the number of errors in the arresting consonant error category for each of the seven high and eight low intelligibility laryngectomized speakers for the PB words, showing x̄, N and σ for each group.

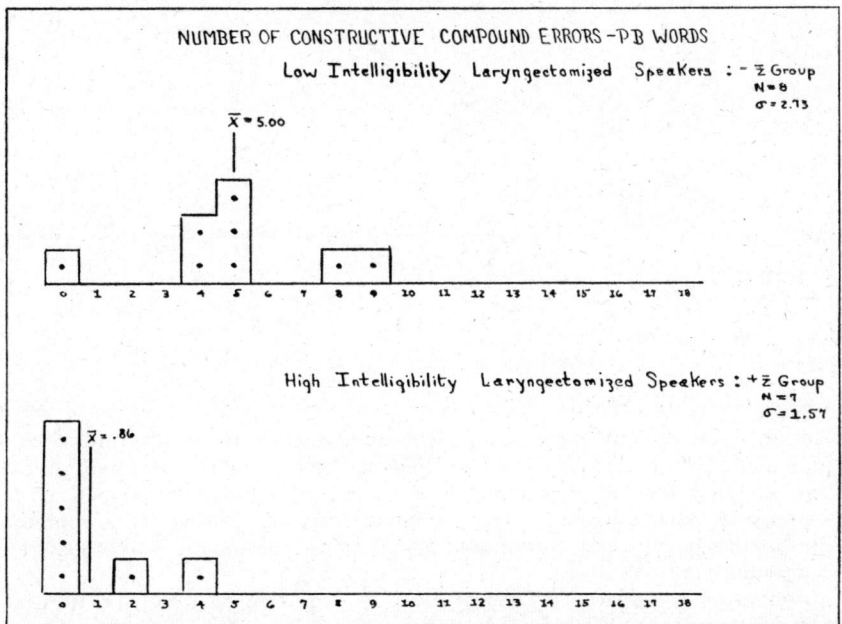

FIG. 55. Distribution of the number of errors in the constructive compound consonant error category for each of the seven high and eight low intelligibility laryngectomized speakers for the PB words, showing x̄, N and σ for each group.

three error categories are significant beyond the .05 level. The t values for the constructive compound and substitution error categories reveal that the difference between means is significant beyond the .01 level. In the vowel error categories only one error category reveals any significant difference between the means. In the neutralization error category the **F** is significant. When the t value is corrected it still remains significant beyond the .05 level. Of the consonant error categories, five of the six categories reveal significant differences between the means.

Evaluation of Rhythm Differences Between High and Low Intelligibility Groups

Table 46 summarizes the rhythm data (total number of sentences spoken with normal rhythm) for the laryngectomized speakers as a

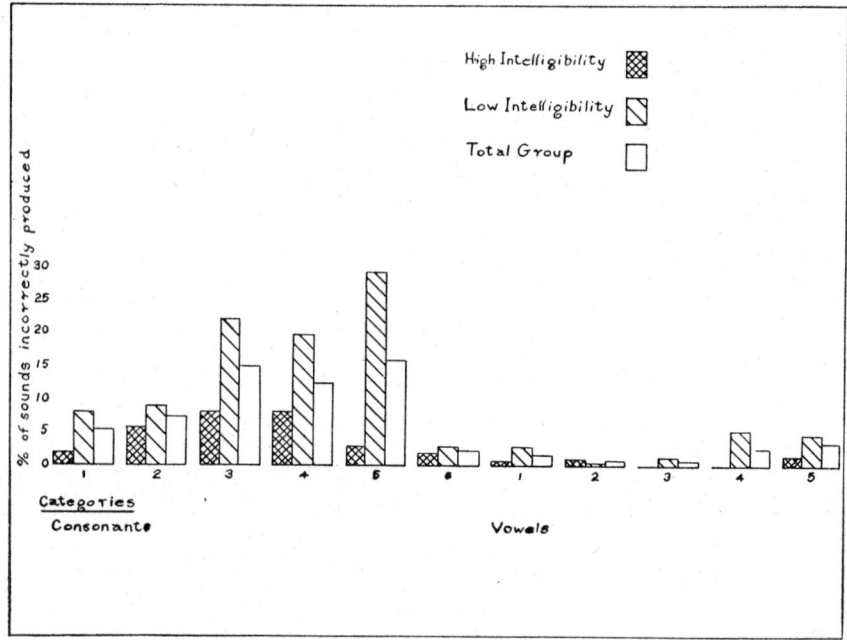

Fig. 56. The percentages of sounds produced incorrectly in the various consonant and vowel error categories for the seven high and eight low intelligibility laryngectomized speakers and for the total group in the sentence material.
Consonant error categories: 1) surd-sonant, 2) substitution, 3) compound consonant, 4) releasing consonant, 5) arresting consonant, 6) constructive compound.
Vowel error categories: 1) substitution, 2) diphthongization, 3) neutralization, 4) omission, 5) constructive release.

group and also broken down into high and low intelligibility groupings. The mean of the total group is 5.40 sentences, but when the speakers are considered in their intelligibility groupings, the high intelligibility group $(+\bar{z})$ has a mean of 8.14 sentences with normal rhythm, while the low intelligibility group $(-\bar{z})$ has a mean of 3.00 sentences. The difference between the means of the two groups on this variable is 5.14, being significant at the .01 level of confidence. This is further evidence of the predictive value of rhythm as an indicator of intelligibility.

Figure 58 illustrates the distribution of sentences spoken with normal rhythm for the low and high intelligibility groups. The difference between the means of the two groups is clearly indicated.

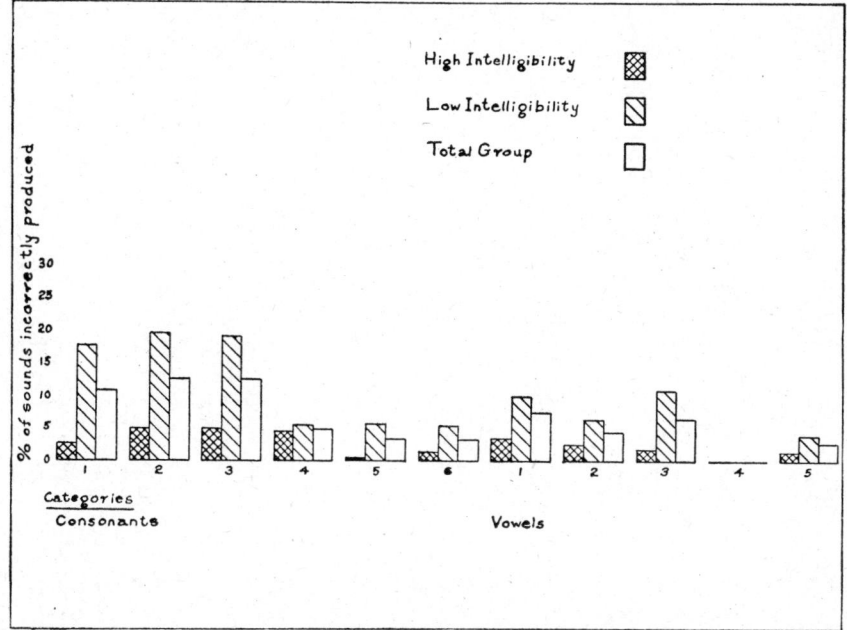

FIG. 57. Percentages of sounds produced incorrectly in the various consonant and vowel error categories for the seven high and eight low intelligibility laryngectomized speakers and for the total group in the PB material.
Consonant error categories: 1) surd-sonant, 2) substitution, 3) compound consonant, 4) releasing consonant, 5) arresting consonant, 6) constructive compound.
Vowel error categories: 1) substitution, 2) diphthongization, 3) neutralization, 4) omission, 5) constructive release.

CORRELATIONS OF INTELLIGIBILITY CRITERIA AND INTELLIGIBILITY PREDICTORS

Analysis of the speech coordination data reveals that two discriminating variables between normal and laryngectomized speakers are total time in speaking a speech sample and the number of phrases employed in speaking this speech sample. Not only do these predictive variables discriminate between the laryngectomized and normal subjects, but they also differentiate between laryngectomized speakers who are considered to be highly intelligible and laryngectomized speakers who are less intelligible. Additional analysis of the recorded speech materials reveals that the variables of articulatory errors and rhythm in the speech of laryngectomized individuals would also discriminate better and poorer speakers. The question then arises concerning the relationships between each predictor variable (rhythm, time, phrases and articulatory errors) with each criterion employed in the study, namely: PB words, multiple choice test and the sentences. In addition

TABLE 45

MEANS, VARIANCES, STANDARD DEVIATIONS, DIFFERENCES BETWEEN THE MEANS, t AND F VALUES AND CORRECTED t WHEN THE F VALUE IS SIGNIFICANT FOR THE CONSONANT AND VOWEL ERROR CATEGORIES FOR PB WORDS FOR THE SEVEN HIGH AND EIGHT LOW INTELLIGITILITY GROUPS OF LARYNGECTOMIZED SPEAKERS

	Variables	High $+\bar{z}$ Group			Low $-\bar{z}$ Group			$\bar{X}_{+\bar{z}}-\bar{X}_{-\bar{z}}$	t	Cal. t .05	F
		$\bar{X}$	σ^2	σ	$\bar{X}$	σ^2	σ				
	Total consonants	9.57	11.29	3.36	39.75	39.93	6.32	30.18	11.28**		3.54
	Total vowels	3.86	6.48	2.54	15.00	61.71	7.86	11.14	3.58**		9.52
Consonants	Surd-sonant	1.57	2.29	1.51	9.38	19.13	4.37	7.80	4.73x	2.38	8.32**
	Substitution	4.57	3.62	1.90	17.88	15.27	3.91	13.30	8.17**		4.22
	Compound consonants	.86	.48	.69	3.38	4.27	2.07	2.52	3.25x	2.37	8.96**
	Releasing consonants	1.57	.95	.98	2.00	3.43	1.85	.43	.55		3.60
	Arresting consonants	.14	.14	.38	2.13	3.84	1.96	1.98	2.80x	2.37	26.87**
	Constructive compound	.86	2.48	1.57	5.00	7.43	2.73	4.14	3.53**		3.00
Vowels	Substitution	1.86	2.48	1.57	5.25	15.08	3.88	3.39	2.15		6.09
	Diphthongization	.86	1.48	1.22	2.25	2.50	1.58	1.39	1.89		1.69
	Neutralization	.57	.29	.53	5.50	22.01	4.69	4.93	2.95x	2.37	76.97**
	Omission	0.00	0.00	0.00	0.00	0.00	0.00	0.00	0.00		0.00
	Constructive release	.57	.62	.79	2.00	3.14	1.77	1.43	1.96		5.08

$df = N_1 + N_2 - 2$
$df = 13$
$t_{.01} = 3.012$
$t_{.05} = 2.160$

** = .01
* = .05

xx = .01 level - Indicates significance of t
x = .05 level when F is significant

df = 7 and 6
$F_{.02} = 8.26$
$F_{.05} = 6.74$
(Interpolated)
$F_{.10} = 4.21$

** = .02
* = .05

the interrelation of the three criteria was investigated. Table 47 is a summary of the data relating to the Pearson r correlations which were determined. Considering correlations of rhythm, time, phrases and consonant and vowel errors with PB intelligibility we find that the r's are significant at the .01 level of confidence with the highest correlation of −.96 for consonant errors with PB's with 92 per cent of predictable variance. Considering the time factor correlated with PB's it proves to have the lowest correlation of the three, of .65 with 42 per cent of predictable variance. The Pearson r for phrases with PB is .74 with a predictable variance of 75 per cent. The multiple choice correlations are .74 for rhythm, with 54 per cent of predictable variance, .50 for time with 25 per cent of predictable variance, and .62 for phrases with 38 per cent of predictable variance. All of these values are lower than the PB correlations with these same variables, but phrases and rhythm continue to be significantly related to the criterion. Finally, the criterion, sentences with rhythm, time, phrases, consonant and vowel errors relate with Pearson r's of .73 with 54 per cent of predictable variance, .70 with 49 per cent of predictable variance, .51 with 26 per cent of predictable variance, −.88 for consonant errors with 77 per cent of predictable variance and −.84 for vowel errors with 71 per cent of predictable variance. Consonant and vowel errors continue to offer the

TABLE 46

MEANS, VARIANCES, STANDARD DEVIATIONS, DIFFERENCE BETWEEN THE MEANS, t AND F VALUES FOR RHYTHM SCORES ON SENTENCES FOR SEVEN HIGH AND EIGHT LOW INTELLIGIBILITY GROUPS OF LARYNGECTOMIZED SPEAKERS

Group	$\overline{X}$	σ^2	σ	$\overline{X}_{+\bar{z}} - \overline{X}_{-\bar{z}}$	t	F
Total group N = 15	5.40	9.54	3.09			
+z̄ group N = 7	8.14	4.14	2.04			
				5.14	6.06**	2.90
−z̄ group N = 8	3.00	1.42	1.20			

** = .01

highest correlations and greatest percentages of predictable variance with rhythm as the next highest variable.

Considering the intercorrelations of the three criteria, we find that the two criteria most closely related are the PB's and multiple choice test with a correlation of .86 significant at the .01 level of confidence, with 74 per cent of predictable variance. The type of material employed in the PB's and the multiple choice test are similar in that there is a minimum of communicative value involved. The PB's are a list of monosyllabic words and the multiple choice test is a series of three one-word phrases. The Pearson r for sentences and multiple choice is .64, significant at the .01 level of confidence, with 41 per cent of predictable variance; and the Pearson r for PB's and sentences is .77, also significant

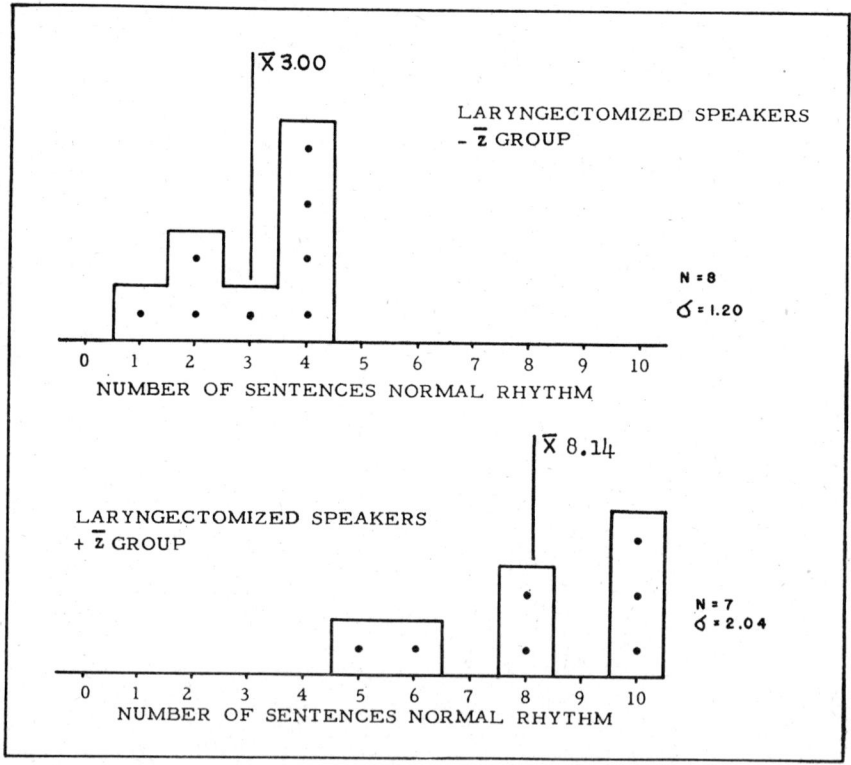

FIG. 58. Distribution of the number of sentences having normal rhythm for the laryngectomized speakers, divided into two groups, (1) those higher than the mean on the combined intelligibility score (+z̄ group), and (2) those lower than the mean on the combined intelligibility score (−z̄ group) indicating x̄, N and σ for the two groups.

at the .01 level of confidence, with 59 per cent of predictable variance (Figure 48). Hudgins (24) reports markedly similar results, a Pearson r of .76 for the relationship between sentences and monosyllabic words (PBF). In addition he applied the correlation ratio method for curvilinear distributions to his data and found a correlation of .81. When this method was applied to the data in the present study, a correlation

TABLE 47

PEARSON'S CORRELATIONS, GIVING INTERCORRELATIONS BETWEEN THE THREE INTELLIGIBILITY SCORES AND THE PREDICTORS: ABDOMINAL AND CHEST AMPLITUDE, TIME AND NUMBER OF PHRASES FOR THE SIXTY-SYLLABLE PARAGRAPH AND THE NUMBER OF RHYTHMICAL SENTENCES FOR THE SENTENCE MATERIAL, AND THE RELATIONSHIP BETWEEN SENTENCE INTELLIGIBILITY SCORES, PB INTELLIGIBILITY SCORES AND CONSONANT AND VOWEL ERRORS AND ERROR CATEGORIES OF SENTENCES AND PB WORDS AS SHOWN BY r, r^2, REGRESSION COEFFICIENTS (b_{yx}) AND STANDARD ERROR OF ESTIMATE ($\sigma_{y.x}$)

		PB Words				Sentences				Multiple Choice			
		r	r^2	b_{yx}	$\sigma_{y.x}$	r	r^2	b_{yx}	$\sigma_{y.x}$	r	r^2	b_{yx}	$\sigma_{y.x}$
Inter-correlation	PB					.7658	.5864	.59	15.61	.8586	.7372	1.35	12.45
	M. C.					.6410	.4109	.31	11.83				
Ampli-tude	Abdominal	-.3029	.0917	-2.04	23.14	-.3257	.1061	-2.86	29.94	-.2950	.0870	-1.26	14.72
	Chest	-.0268	.0007	-.14	24.27	-.2683	.0720	-1.85	30.51	-.1988	.0395	-.67	15.10
Variables Used in Predicting Intelligibility	Time	-.6511	.4239	-.54	18.43	-.7024	.4934	-.76	22.54	-.5041	.2541	-.26	13.31
	Phrases	-.7460	.5565	-1.12	16.17	-.5141	.2643	-1.01	27.16	-.6204	.3849	-.59	12.09
	Rhythm	.8343	.6961	6.55	1.70	.7341	.5389	7.52	2.10	.7378	.5443	3.68	2.09
Total Consonants	Sentences	-.8639	.7463	-1.54	12.23	-.8790	.7726	-2.05	15.10				
	PB	-.9569	.9157	-1.42	7.05	-.8280	.6858	-1.60	17.75				
Total Vowels	Sentences	-.7773	.6041	-3.40	15.28	-.8437	.7118	-4.81	17.00				
	PB	-.7196	.5178	-2.14	16.86	-.7830	.6131	-3.03	19.70				
Sentences Consonants	Surd-sonant	-.8016	.6425	-8.73	14.52	-.6013	.3615	-8.54	25.31				
	Substitution	-.5242	.2727	-2.63	20.71	-.1249	.0160	-.82	31.42				
	Compound consonant	-.4286	.1836	-4.60	21.94	-.4501	.2025	-6.31	28.28				
	Releasing consonant	-.4421	.1954	-2.12	21.78	-.7871	.6189	-4.92	19.55				
	Arresting consonant	-.7179	.5153	-3.21	16.90	-.8796	.7726	-5.13	15.10				
	Constructive compound	-.0788	.0062	-.51	24.20	-.0583	.0033	-.49	31.62				
PB Consonants	Surd-sonant	-.7508	.5637	-3.53	16.04	-.6229	.3880	-3.82	24.78				
	Substitution	-.9077	.8239	-2.93	10.19	-.7758	.6019	-3.27	19.98				
	Compound consonant	-.7059	.4983	-8.53	17.20	-.7804	.6090	-12.30	19.80				
	Releasing consonant	-.2757	.0760	-4.55	23.34	-.4336	.1880	-9.34	28.54				
	Arresting consonant	-.5830	.3399	-8.14	19.73	-.5418	.2927	-9.85	26.63				
	Constructive compound	-.6919	.4787	-5.49	17.53	-.4418	.1952	-4.57	28.41				
Sentences Vowels	Substitution	-.5275	.2782	-7.12	20.63	-.7184	.5160	-12.64	22.03				
	Diphthongization	-.0800	.0064	-4.22	24.20	.2058	.0423	14.17	30.99				
	Neutralization	-.6517	.4247	-24.72	18.42	-.1063	.0112	-5.26	31.49				
	Omission	-.5890	.3469	-4.72	19.62	-.9129	.8333	-9.54	12.93				
	Constructive-release	-.4949	.2449	-5.20	21.10	-.0892	.0079	-1.22	31.54				
PB Vowels	Substitution	-.5154	.2656	-3.66	20.81	-.7702	.5932	-7.13	20.20				
	Diphthongization	-.3710	.1376	-5.81	22.55	-.2519	.0635	-5.15	30.65				
	Neutralization	-.7005	.4913	-4.05	17.32	-.7063	.4989	-5.33	22.42				
	Omission	.0	.0			.0	.0						
	Constructive-release	-.3907	.1526	-6.16	22.35	-.2670	.0713	-5.49	30.52				

df = 13
** r .01 = .641
* r .05 = .514

Significance for Pearson r found in Snedecor's, *Statistical Methods*, Ames, Iowa: Iowa State College Press, 1946, Table 13.6, p. 351.

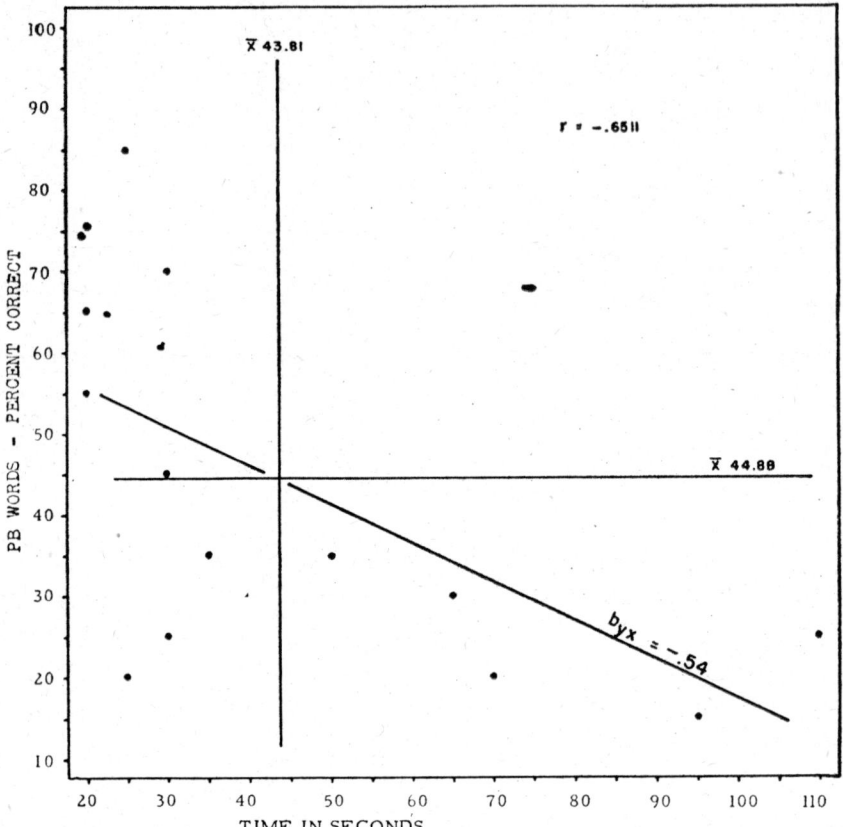

Fɪɢ. 59. Scatter diagram indicating relationship between the intelligibility criterion PB words in per cent correct and the predictor total time in speaking the sixty-syllable paragraph by the laryngectomized individuals, showing means, regression line and Pearson r.

of .93 was found. The relationship between PB and sentences has also been reported by Eagan (14).

Figures 59, 60 and 61 are scatter diagrams revealing the relationship of the PB's with time, phrases, and rhythm.

Figures 62, 63 and 64 reveal the relationship between the multiple choice intelligibility test and time, phrases and rhythm.

Figures 65, 66 and 67 are scatter diagrams revealing the relationship of sentences to time, phrases, and rhythm.

Figures 68 through 70 reveal the relationships between the criteria, multiple choice intelligibility test, sentences, and PB's.

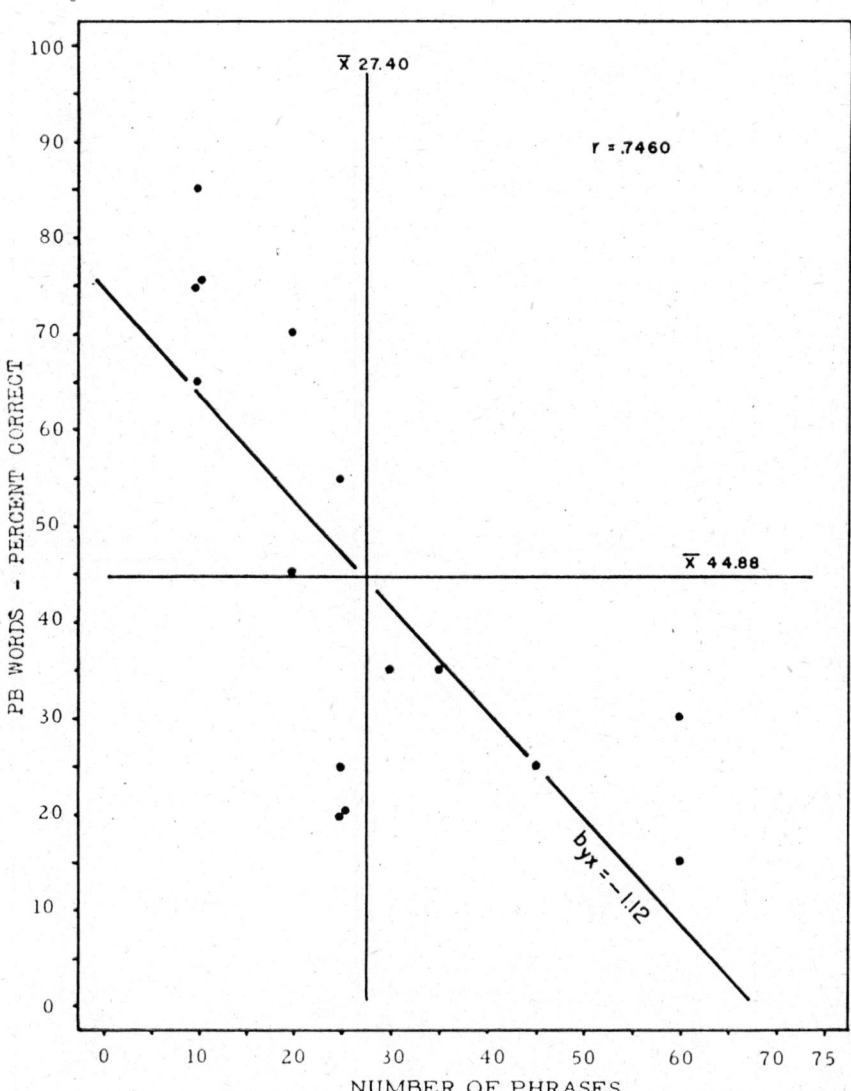

Fig. 60. Scatter diagram indicating relationship between the intelligibility criterion, PB words in per cent correct, and the predictor, number of phrases used in speaking the sixty-syllable paragraph by the laryngectomized individuals, showing means, regression line and Pearson r.

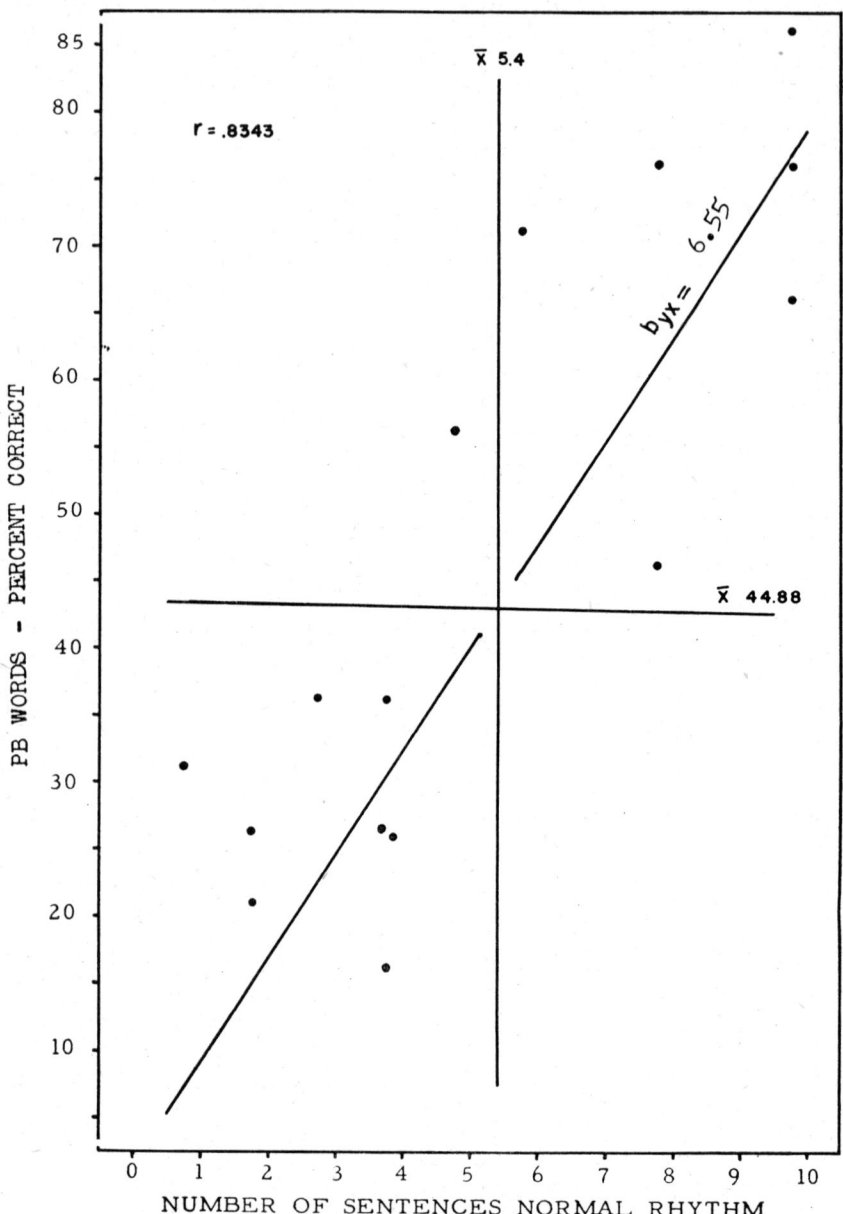

FIG. 61. Scatter diagram indicating relationship between the intelligibility criterion PB words in per cent correct and the predictor number of sentences spoken with normal rhythm by the laryngectomized individuals showing means, regression line and Pearson r.

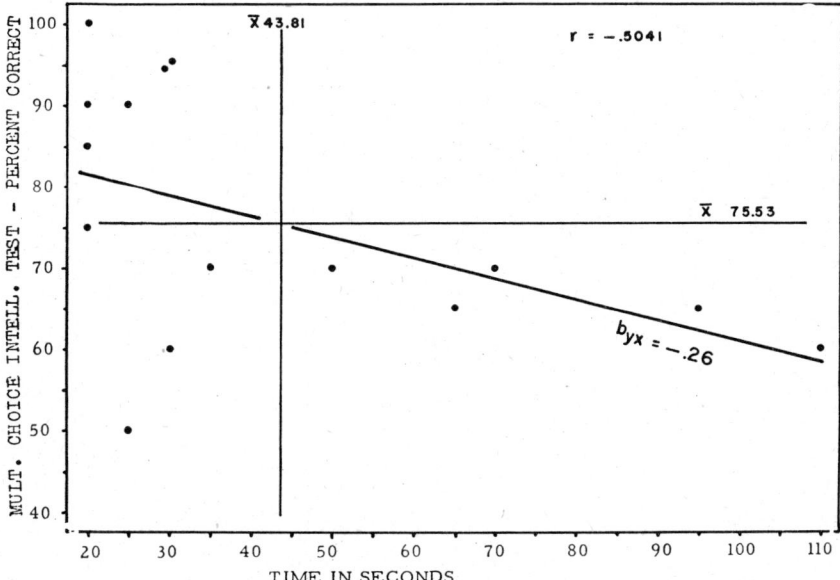

Fig. 62. Scatter diagram indicating relationship between the intelligibility criterion, multiple choice test, in per cent words correct and predictor, total time, in seconds in speaking the sixty-syllable paragraph by the laryngectomized individuals, showing means, regression line and Pearson r.

Table 47 also reveals that the correlations for total consonant and total vowel categories with sentence intelligibility are —.88 with 77 per cent of predictable variance for the consonants, while the correlation is —.84 with a percentage of predictable variance of 71 for vowels. This would indicate that both vowel and consonant errors are of approximately equal importance in sentence intelligibility. In the consonant error categories contributing toward sentence intelligibility, the arresting, releasing and the surd-sonant show significant relationships at either the .05 or .01 level of confidence. The correlations reveal that the arresting consonant category is highly related to intelligibility with an r of —.88 and a predictable variance of 77 per cent. The percentage of predictable variance for the releasing consonant is .62. Further analysis of the table reveals that these three categories are significantly related to speech intelligibility for the sentence material. For the vowels, omission and substitution appear to contribute most heavily toward intelligibility with correlations of —.91 and —.72 with predictable variance of 83 per cent and 52 per cent respectively. The relationship between the consonant errors and PB intelligibility scores show a

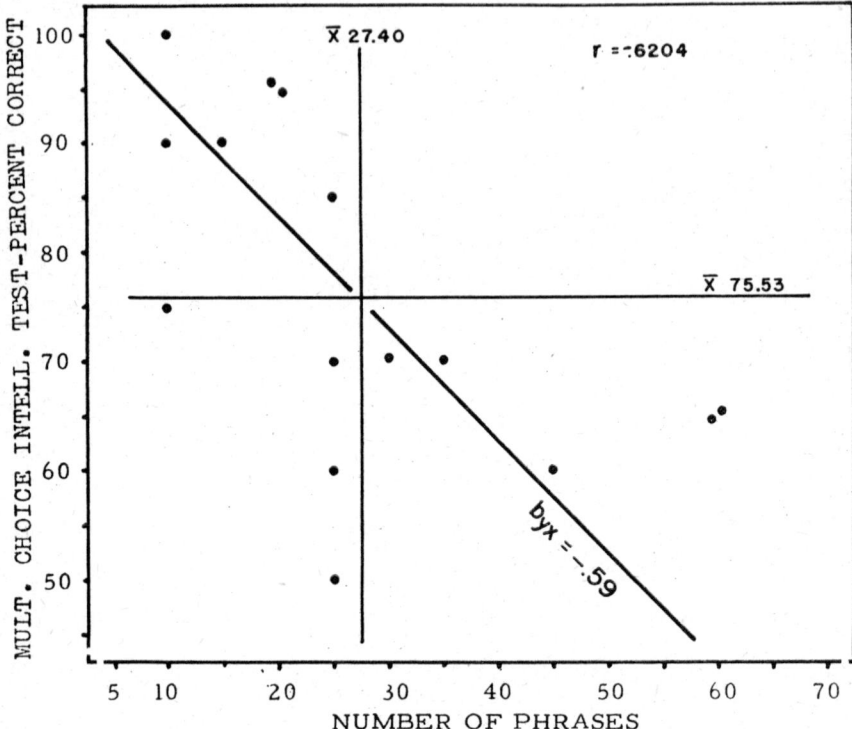

Fig. 63. Scatter diagram indicating relationship between the intelligibility criterion, multiple choice test, in per cent of words correct and the predictor, number of phrases, in speaking the sixty-syllable paragraph by the laryngectomized individuals, showing means, regression line and Pearson r.

similar relationship with a slightly lower correlation and percentage of predictable variance for the vowels. The table also reveals that the surd-sonant and arresting consonants remain significant for the sentence and PB materials. The relationship changes with respect to releasing consonants. For the sentence materials the releasing consonant is significant beyond the .01 level, while it does not prove to be significant for the PB's. On the other hand, while the substitution category for the sentences is not significant, it acquires significance at better than the .05 level for PB's. The table also indicates that for the vowels, substitution and omission are significant for both materials. Neutralization does not prove to be significant in the sentences but attains significance at better than the .01 level for the PB's. For the sentence material, the surd-sonant, releasing, arresting consonants, and sub-

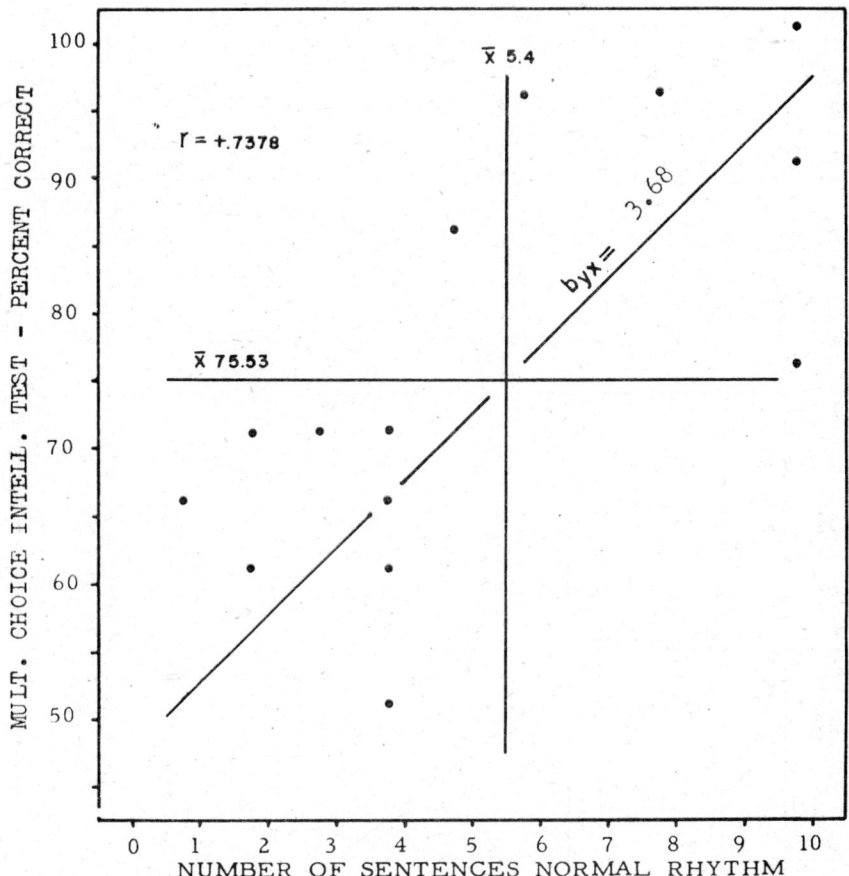

Fig. 64. Scatter diagram indicating relationship between the intelligibility criterion, multiple choice test, in per cent of words correct and the predictor, number of sentences spoken, with normal rhythm, showing means, regression line and Pearson r.

stitution and omission for the vowels prove to be significant. In the sentence, "The window measured four feet wide," some laryngectomized speakers did not make the surd-sonant distinction in the word "wide," and some auditors heard it as "white." Others heard the arresting "t" but could not identify the vowel and understood the word as "wet." In both of these cases the total sentence was incorrect because the word "white" and "wet" could not fit into any meaningful framework. In the sentence, "The cab stopped at his house," the speaker left off [ð] and most of the auditors heard the [ðɑ] as [hi] and others omitted the word.

In this case the sentence could not be guessed at because the beginning words would not permit possibility of meaning in context. In the sentence, "He walked to the hotel," the [h] was omitted in the word "hotel," and some of the auditors heard the word as "order." In both cases the releasing error contributed to the unintelligibility of the sentence. In the sentence, "The motor of the car was defective," the speaker did not give the arresting [v] its proper coordination and the auditors heard the word as "confessed," "unfed," "fastened." The inability to attribute meaning to this last word did not permit meaning for the entire sentence.

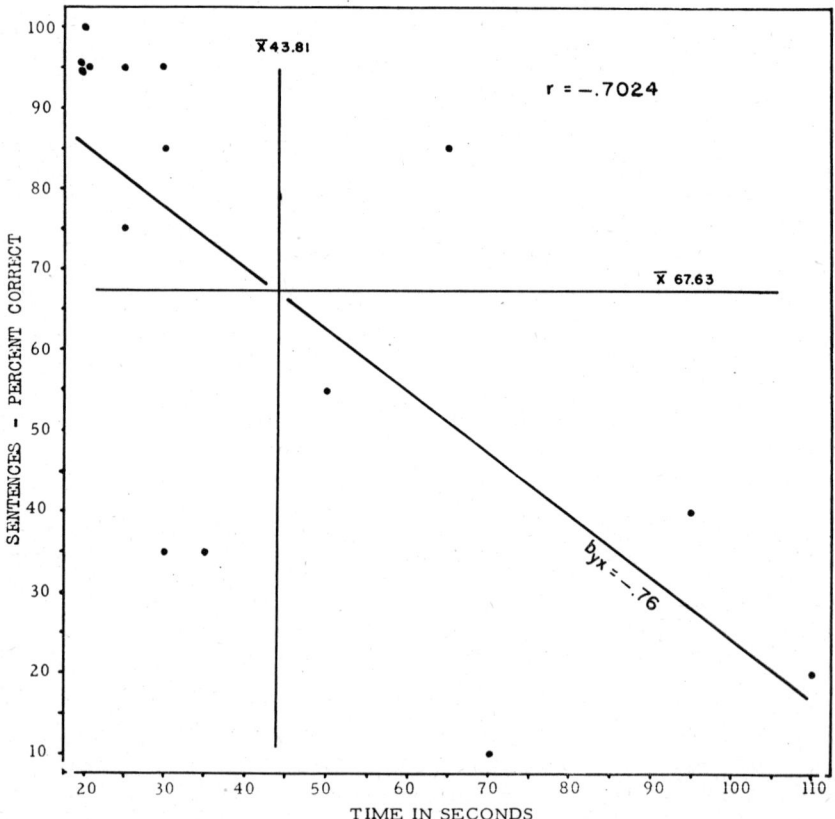

FIG. 65. Scatter diagram indicating the relationship between the intelligibility criterion, sentences per cent correct, and the predictor, total time in seconds, in speaking the sixty-syllable paragraph for the laryngectomized individuals showing means, regression line and Pearson r.

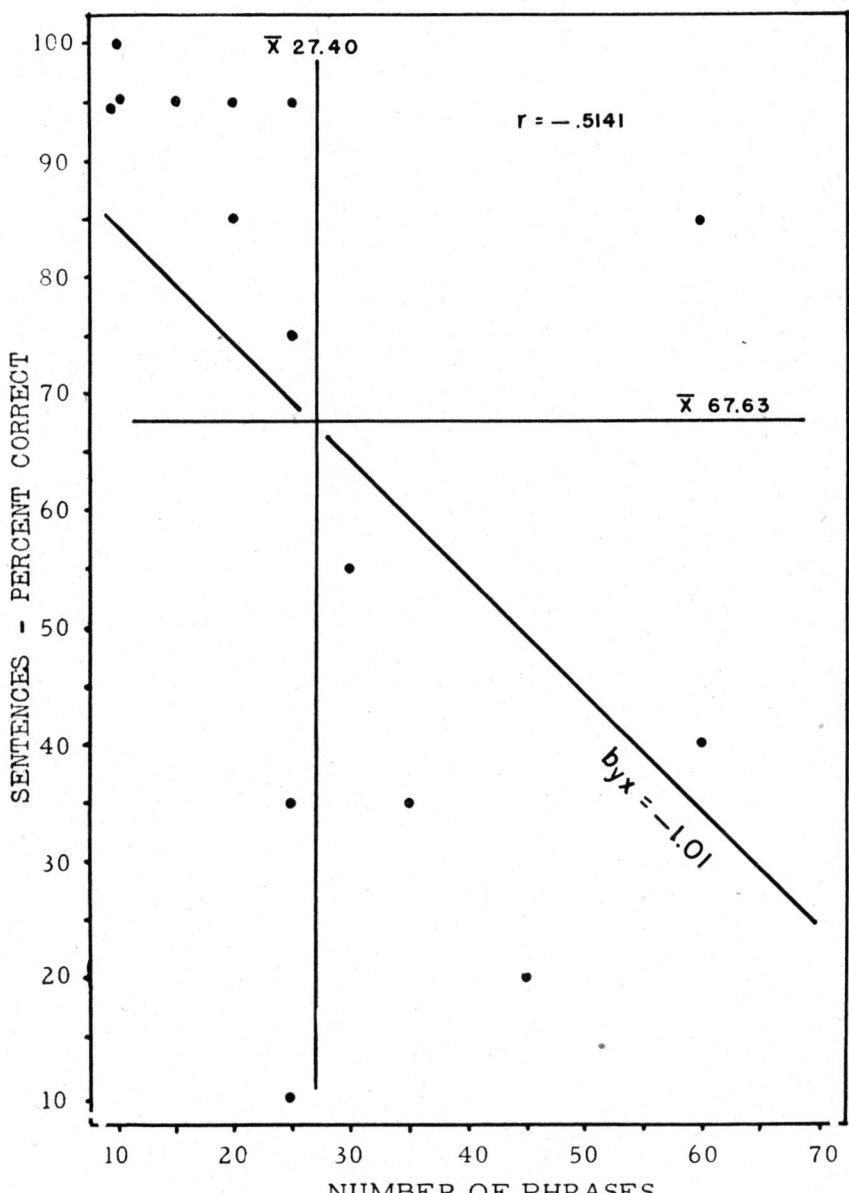

Fig. 66. Scatter diagram indicating the relationship between the intelligibility criterion, sentences per cent correct, and the predictor, number of phrases, in speaking the sixty-syllable paragraph for the laryngectomized individuals showing means, regression line and Pearson r.

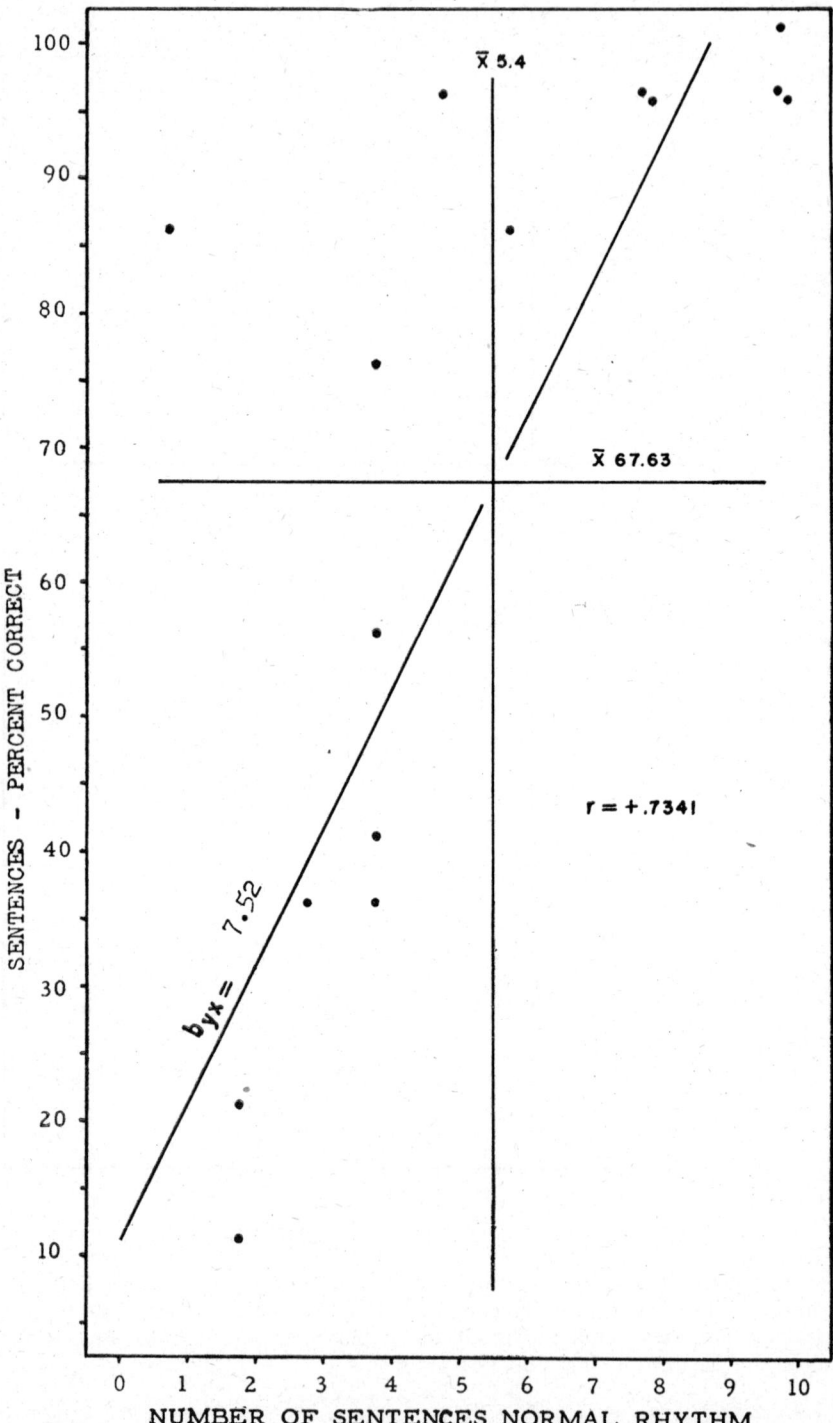

Fig. 67. Scatter diagram indicating the relationship between the intelligibility criterion, sentences, per cent correct, and the predictor, number of sentences spoken with normal rhythm, showing means, regression line and Pearson r.

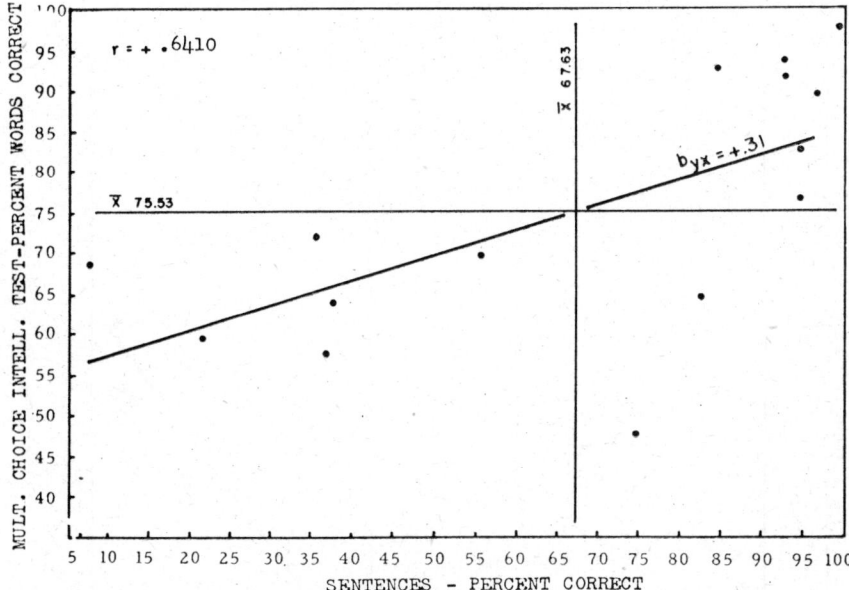

FIG. 68. Scatter diagram indicating the relationship between two intelligibility criteria, multiple choice test, per cent of words correct and sentences, per cent correct, showing means, regression line, and Pearson r.

Table 47 further shows the relationship between PB intelligibility, sentence intelligibility and consonant and vowel error categories. The correlations for consonant errors with PB intelligibility is −.96 with 92 per cent of predictable variance, and for vowel errors the correlation is −.72 with a percentage of predictable variance of 52. The correlations are significant at better than the .01 level. For the sentence material, three of the six consonant categories are significant, but five of the consonant categories for the PB materials are significant, indicating that practically all of the categories are necessary for intelligibility since monosyllabic words do not offer contextual cues. For both sentence and PB materials, two vowel error categories are significant. Apparently vowel errors do not contribute as much to intelligibility as consonant errors.

In the PB word "pack" the laryngectomized individual spoke it as "plack." In this he virtually constructed a compound out of a single releasing plosive. Of six auditors, one understood him as "back," two as "black," one as "pack" and two as "plack." In the word "leave" the individual spoke it as "glif." In this case he constructed a constructive

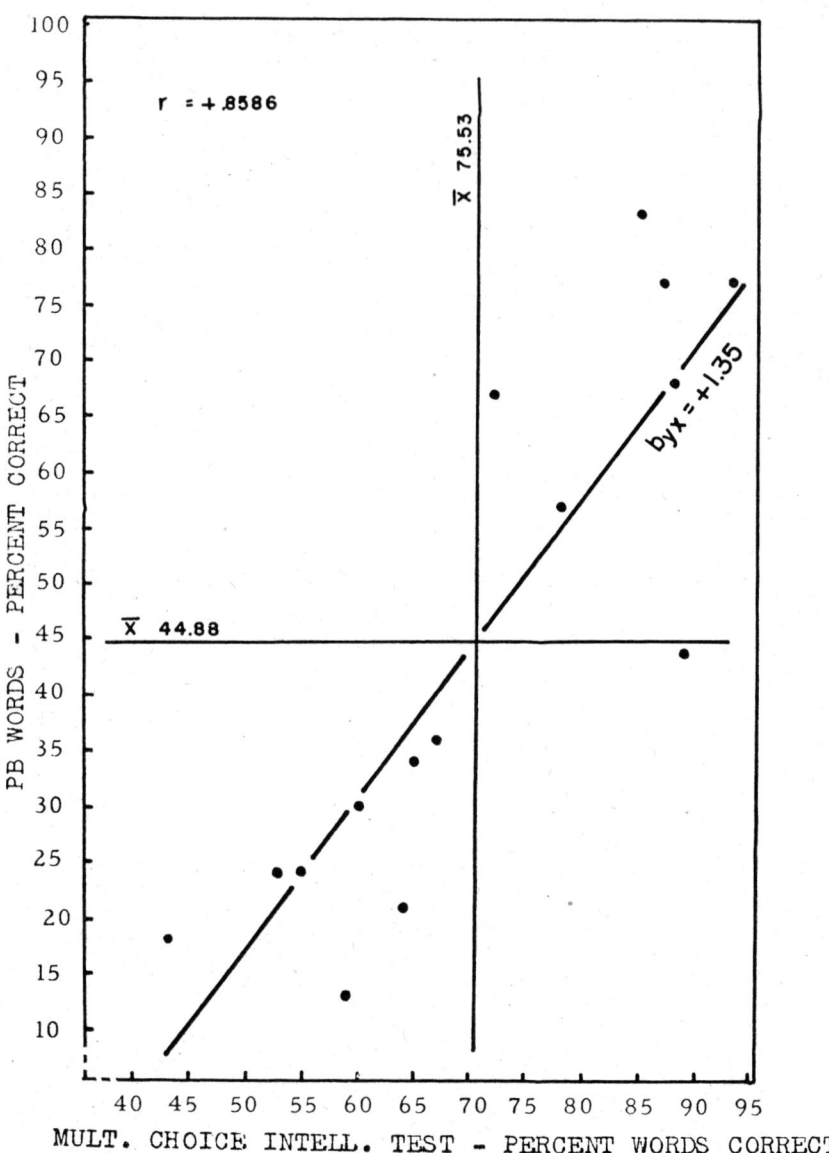

Fig. 69. Scatter diagram indicating the relationship between two intelligibility criteria, PB words per cent correct and multiple choice test per cent of words correct, showing means, regression line and Pearson r.

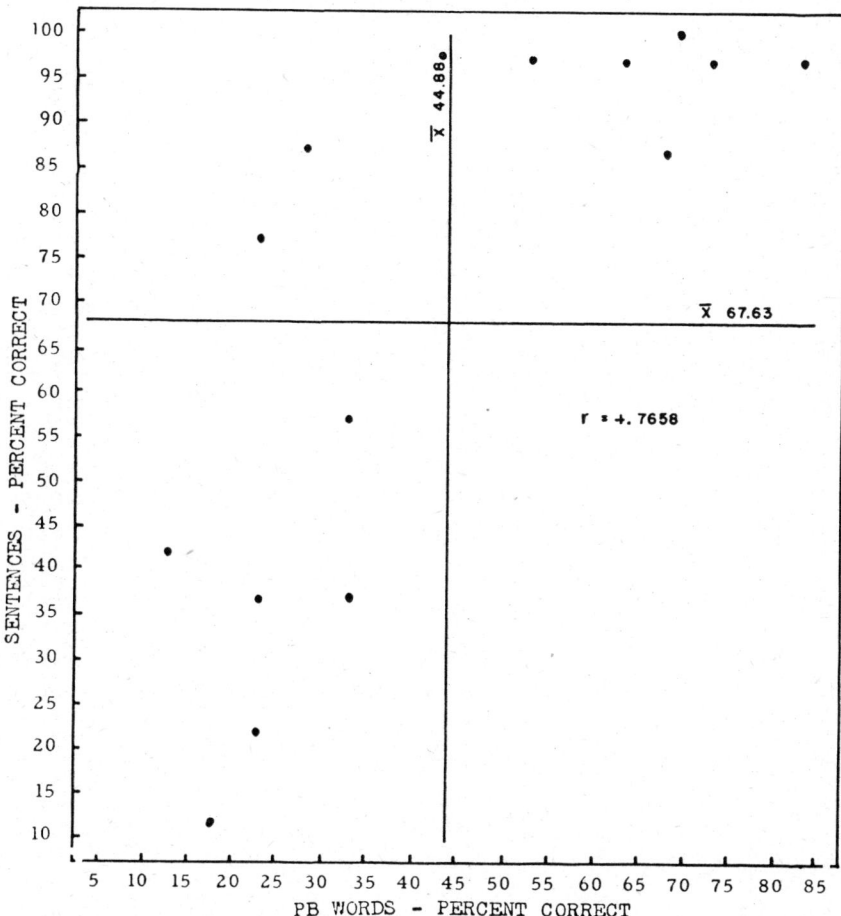

FIG. 70. Scatter diagram indicating the relationship between two intelligibility criteria, sentences, per cent correct, and PB words, per cent correct, showing means, and Pearson r.

compound and did not make the surd-sonant distinction. The six auditors heard him as "glich," "lead," "glig," "chick," "live" and "blade." These examples indicate that the integrity of the word must be preserved in order to permit meaning. Where meaning is involved the consonants and vowels must be more correctly articulated in mono-syllabic material than in sentence material where contextual cues will help the auditor. This tendency to construct compounds especially in the releasing position is more evident in the low intelligibility speakers.

Examination of the samples reveals that for the PB materials less distortion would be permitted. When considering intelligibility, both sentence and PB, in relation to the predictors examined in the study, consonant errors offer the highest correlations and the greatest percentages of predictable variance.

RELATIONSHIP OF INTELLIGIBILITY WITH SEVERAL VARIABLES

Examination of the data raises an additional question as to what combinations of the predictor variables would yield highest correlation and offer most predictive information. Table 48 is a matrix of the Pearson r's used to implement the multiple correlation analysis. Table 49 is a summary of the multiple correlation data. The table reveals the relationships of the multiple choice test to the combinations of rhythm and time, and rhythm and phrases, and time and phrases. We observe that the multiple r's of .7389 for rhythm and time and .7397 for rhythm and phrases approximate the Pearson r of rhythm and multiple choice .7378. For the PB's; rhythm and time, and rhythm and phrases, both indicate higher correlations with higher percentages of predictable variance than for the combination of time and phrases. The multiple r values for rhythm and time and rhythm and phrases are almost identical, being .8479 and .8448 respectively. At this point it is evident that rhythm alone with PB's has contributed as much percentage of predictable variance as the combination of rhythm and time or rhythm and phrases. In predicting PB intelligibility from the different two

TABLE 48

INTERCORRELATION MATRIX OF PEARSON r's FOR THE FIVE PREDICTORS: RHYTHM, TIME, PHRASES, CONSONANT ERRORS (SENTENCE AND PB) AND VOWEL ERRORS IN SENTENCES, AND THREE CRITERION VARIABLES: PB LISTS, MULTIPLE CHOICE TESTS AND SENTENCES

Variables N = 15	Predictors					Criteria		
	Rhythm	Time	Phrases	Consonants Sentences	PB	Intelligibility PB	Sentence	Multiple Choice
Rhythm		-.6409*	-.7982**	-.7211***	-.7985***	.8343***	.7341***	.7378***
Time	-.6409*		.7816***	.7823***	.6572**	-.6511**	-.7024***	-.5041
Phrases	-.7982**	.7816***		.6278*	.6834***	-.7460***	-.5141*	-.6204*
Consonants Sentences	-.7211***	.7823***	.6278*			-.8639***	-.8790***	
Consonants PB	-.7985***	.6572**	.6834***			-.9569***	-.8280**	
Vowels	-.7498***	.7913***	.5990*	.8463***			-.7830***	

$$r_{.01} = .641$$
$$r_{.05} = .514$$

predictor combinations of consonant errors, rhythm, time and phrases, the values for the combinations do not differ greatly from the relationship shown by the Pearson r for consonant errors with PB intelligibility (−.9569) with 91.57 per cent of predictable variance. When the three and four predictor correlations are computed, the values do not change greatly and do not offer appreciably greater predictable variance than the Pearson r for consonant errors with PB intelligibility. For example, the combination of rhythm-time-phrases and consonant errors with PB intelligibility yielded the largest multiple r, .9681, with 93.72 per cent of predictable variance. This afforded only a 2.15 per cent increase in predictable variance over the value afforded when relating consonant errors with PB intelligibility.

With respect to the criterion, sentences, the multiple r for rhythm and time, .7939, increased somewhat over the Pearson r, .7341, for rhythm and sentences, and the per cent of predictable variance increased from 54 to approximately 63 per cent. When predicting sentence intelligibility from the different two predictor combinations of consonant errors and rhythm, time and phrases, the correlations do not increase appreciably and do not offer sufficiently greater predictive information than when consonant errors alone are related to sentence intelligibility, (Pearson r −.8790 with 77.26 per cent of predictable variance). When the three predictor correlations are computed, two of the correlations remain essentially the same and two increase slightly. When the four predictor correlation is computed, the correlation increases from −.88 with a predictable variance of 77 per cent to .92 with a percentage of predictable variance of 85. When the one criterion five predictor correlation is computed, it does not increase the correlation appreciably above the four predictor situation. Examination of Table 49 further reveals that for the sentence material there is an increase in the correlation when additional predictors are included. The variables, time, phrases and rhythm, contribute to intelligibility in addition to consonant and vowel errors. For the PB material the correlation coefficients are not improved when additional variables are included. For the monosyllabic words consonant errors permit greatest predictive information.

Analysis of the different consonant error categories for both sentences and PB material suggests that for the sentence material certain combinations of error categories may contribute more to intelligibility than other combinations. Table 50 reveals the relationship of multiples of three consonant error categories with sentence intelligibility. When combinations of surd-sonant, releasing and arresting consonants appear, the correlation coefficient should be high, since the correlation coefficient for each individual category with intelligibility is high. Table 50 shows the correlation coefficient for the three highest, surd-sonant, arresting and releasing consonants. This coefficient is .94 which is significant at better than the .01 level with a percentage of predictable variance of .88. When the three lowest, compound consonant, constructive compound and substitution error categories are related to intelligibility, the correlation is .47, which is not significant. When two highs

TABLE 49

MULTIPLE r, r^2 AND k^2 FOR THE THREE CRITERION VARIABLES: PB LISTS, MULTIPLE CHOICE TEST AND SENTENCES, AND FOUR PREDICTORS OF TIME, RHYTHM, PHRASES AND CONSONANT ERRORS (SENTENCE AND PB ERRORS) IN COMBINATIONS OF TWO, THREE AND FOUR PREDICTORS WITH F FOR SIGNIFICANCE OF r^2 AND INCLUDING THE REGRESSION COEFFICIENTS (β WEIGHTS) WITH t FOR TESTING SIGNIFICANCE OF β's

		$r_{o.1...n}$	$r^2_{o.1...n}$	$k^2_{o.1...n}$	$F_{n(N-n-1)}$ [++] $H_0:r^2=0$	β_1	$H_0:\beta_1=0$ t [##]	β_2	$H_0:\beta_2=0$ t	β_3	$H_0:\beta_3=0$ t	β_4	$H_0:\beta_4=0$ t	β_5
Multiple Choice	TP	.6211	.3858	.6142	3.77	-.0493	.13	-.5818	1.57					
	RT	.7389	.5460	.4540	7.22**	.7038	2.78*	-.0530	.21					
	RP	.7397	.5471	.4529	7.25**	.6685	2.07	-.0868	.27					
	RTP	.7397	.5472	.4528	4.43*	.6676	1.98	-.0201	.06	-.0718	.17			
PB Lists	TP	.7539	.5684	.4316	7.90**	.1748	.57	-.6094	2.00					
	RT	.8479	.7190	.2810	15.35**	.7077	3.55**	-.1975	.99					
	RP	.8448	.7137	.2863	14.96**	.6582	2.57*	-.2206	.86					
	RTP	.8497	.7220	.2780	9.52**	.6513	2.47*	-.1463	.57	-.1117	.34			
Consonant Errors	RC	.9162	.8393	.1607	31.34**	.4403	2.64*	-.5464	3.27**					
	TC	.8649	.7480	.2520	17.81**	.0637	.27	-.9138	3.93**					
	PC	.9027	.8148	.1852	26.40**	-.3361	2.11	-.6529	4.09**					
	RTC	.9211	.8485	.1515	20.54**	.4652	2.70*	.1559	.81	-.6504	3.07*			
	RPC	.9203	.8469	.1531	20.28**	.3363	1.52	-.1444	.73	-.5308	3.09*			
	TPC	.9354	.8750	.1250	25.67**	.4919	2.30*	-.5719	3.34**	-.8897	5.19**			
	RTPC	.9410	.8855	.1145	19.33**	.2051	.96	.4184	1.84	-.4197	1.80	-.7798	3.78**	
Consonant Errors	RC	.9640	.9293	.0707	78.87**	.1938	1.51	-.8022	6.29**					
	TC	.9573	.9165	.0835	65.86**	-.0391	.35	-.9312	8.41**					
	PC	.9652	.9316	.0684	81.72**	-.1727	1.67	-.8389	8.11**					
	RTC	.9640	.9293	.0707	48.20**	.1938	1.41	.0005	.04	-.8025	5.72**			
	RPC	.9666	.9344	.0656	52.23**	.1096	.70	-.1208	.93	-.7868	6.09**			
	TPC	.9670	.9350	.0650	52.74**	.0977	.76	-.2338	1.77	-.8613	7.87**			
	RTPC	.9681	.9372	.0650	37.31**	.0948	.58	.0866	.65	-.1817	1.12	-.8140	5.85**	
Sentence Intelligibility	TP	.7046	.4965	.5035	5.92*	-.7725	1.74	.0897	.20					
	RT	.7939	.6302	.3698	10.23**	-.4819	2.11*	-.3936	1.72					
	RP	.7437	.5531	.4468	7.43**	.8922	2.74*	-.1980	.61					
	RTP	.8734	.7629	.2371	11.80**	.8577	3.52**	-.7350	3.12**	.7449	2.48*			
Consonant Errors Sentences	RC	.8908	.7936	.2064	23.07**	.2090	1.10	-.7283	3.85**					
	TC	.8793	.7732	.2268	20.46**	-.0381	.17	-.8492	3.02**					
	PC	.8803	.7749	.2251	20.66**	.0622	.35	-.9180	5.22**					
	RTC	.8908	.7936	.2064	14.10**	.2094	1.04	.0033	.01	-.7306	2.95*			
	RPC	.9096	.8274	.1726	17.58**	.4302	1.83	.3076	1.47	-.7619	4.18**			
	TPC	.8828	.7794	.2206	12.95**	-.1321	.47	.1257	.55	-.8546	3.75**			
	RTC	.9221	.8502	.1498	14.19**	.5313	2.18	-.3218	1.24	.5194	1.94	-.5702	2.42*	
	RTPCV	.9231	.8525	.1475	10.40	.4686		-.2541		.4642		-.5353		-.1163
Consonant Errors PB	RC	.8368	.7003	.2997	14.02**	.2013	.77	-.6673	2.54*					
	TC	.8542	.7296	.2704	16.19**	-.2785	1.40	-.6449	3.24**					
	PC	.8310	.6906	.3094	13.39**	.0971	.44	-.8944	4.07**					
	RTC	.8571	.7346	.2654	10.15**	.1198	.45	-.2541	1.19	-.5654	2.08			
	RPC	.8542	.7297	.2703	9.90**	.4014	1.26	.2872	1.09	-.7037	2.68*			
	TPC	.8895	.7912	.2088	13.89**	-.5282	2.30*	.4265	1.80	-.7723	3.94**			
	RTPC	.9226	.8511	.1489	14.29**	.5011	2.00	-.5856	2.85*	.6998	2.80*	-.5213	2.43*	

	$t_{.01}$	$t_{.05}$
2 Predictors t_{12}	3.055	2.179
3 Predictors t_{11}	3.106	2.201
4 Predictors t_{10}	3.169	2.228

df = N-n-1

n = Number of predictors
N = Number in sample

	$F_{.01}$	$F_{.05}$
2 Predictors F_{2-12}	6.93	3.88
3 Predictors F_{3-11}	6.22	3.59
4 Predictors F_{4-10}	5.99	3.48

df = n, (N-n-1)

[++] Formula 1237 from Truman Lee Kelley, Fundamentals of Statistics. Cambridge, Massachusetts: Harvard University Press, 1947, p. 475.
[##] Formula 14.22 from Palmer O. Johnson, Statistical Methods in Research. New York: Prentice Hall, 1949, p. 339.

and one low are computed, arresting, releasing and constructive compound, the correlation coefficient is .94, which is significant at better than the .01 level with a predictable variance of 88 per cent. When two lows and one high, releasing, constructive compound and substitution, are related to intelligibility, the correlation coefficient is .85, which is lower than .94 but still is significant at better than the .01 level with a predictable variance of 72 per cent. These correlations suggest that in sentence intelligibility the surd-sonant, arresting and releasing consonants contribute a great deal to intelligibility and that when any one

TABLE 50

RELATIONSHIP OF MULTIPLES OF THREE CONSONANT ERROR CATEGORIES[a] WITH SENTENCE INTELLIGIBILITY

	Multiple Error Categories	Sentences r	Intelligibility r^2
3 Highest	Surd-sonant Arresting consonant Releasing consonant	.9389**	.8756
3 Lowest	Compound consonant Constructive compound Substitution	.4679	.2190
2 High and 1 Low	Arresting consonant Releasing consonant Constructive compound	.9360**	.8762
2 Low and 1 High	Releasing consonant Constructive compound Substitution	.8459**	.7156

Significance levels:

3 predictors 4 variables

df = 11 $r_{.01}$** = .793
$r_{.05}$** = .703

[a]Consonant errors in sentence material.

of the three is related with two lows, the correlation is still high. Throughout the study the variables, consonant errors, rhythm, time and phrases, have not only differentiated laryngectomized speakers from normal speakers, but have also differentiated among the laryngectomized speakers. This analysis leads to a further question, the determination of which variable, consonant errors, rhythm, phrases or

TABLE 51

REGRESSION COEFFICIENTS (β WEIGHTS) FOR PREDICTING EACH OF THE THREE INTELLIGIBILITY VARIABLES, PB, MULTIPLE CHOICE AND SENTENCES, FROM COMBINATION OF TWO, THREE AND FOUR OF THE PREDICTORS, RHYTHM, TIME, PHRASES AND CONSONANT ERRORS (SENTENCE AND PB ERRORS) SHOWING F RATIOS FOR SIGNIFICANCE OF DIFFERENCES BETWEEN β's FOR DIRECTION AND ABSOLUTE

		β_1	β_2	β_3	β_4	Direction $F_{\beta_1-\beta_2}$ df=1&12	Absolute $F|\beta_1|-|\beta_2|$ df=1&12	Direction $F_{\beta_1-\beta_3}$	Absolute $F|\beta_1|-|\beta_3|$
Multiple Choice Intelligibility	TP	-.0493	-.5818				.60		
	RT	.7038	-.0530			2.72	2.01		
	RP	.6685	-.0868			1.52	.90		
	RTP	.6676	-.0201	-.0718		2.26	2.00	4.88*	3.17
PB Intelligibility	TP	.1748	-.6094				.57		
	RT	.7077	-.1975			6.28*	2.00		
	RP	.6582	-.2206			3.27*	.81		
	RTP	.6513	-.1463	-.1117		4.94*	1.98	8.46*	4.23
Consonant Errors Sentences	RC	.4403	-.5464			62.61***	.72		
	TC	.0637	-.9138			4.95*	3.75		
	PC	-.3361	-.6529				1.21		
	RTC	.4652	.1559	-.6504			1.75	30.32***	.84
	RPC	.3363	-.1444	-.5308		7.21*	1.15	17.51***	.88
	TPC	.4919	-.5719	-.8897		9.53*	.05	16.04***	1.33
	RTPC	.2051	.4184	-.4197	-.7798		.35	12.00***	1.42
Consonant Errors PB	RC	.1938	-.8022			151.40***	56.49***		
	TC	-.0391	-.9312				19.59***		
	PC	-.1727	-.8389				12.33***		
	RTC	.1938	.0005	-.8025			1.60	73.75***	27.53***
	RPC	.1096	-.1208	-.7868		2.95	.006	44.75***	25.54***
	TPC	.0977	-.2338	-.8613		2.02	.34	25.60***	16.23***
	RTPC	.0948	.0866	-.1817	-.8140		.001	3.18	.31
Sentence Intelligibility	TP	-.7725	.0897			1.06	.67		
	RT	.4819	-.3936			4.47	.05		
	RP	.8922	.1980				1.31		
	RTP	.8577	-.7350	.7449		23.09***	.14		.22
Consonant Errors Sentences	RC	.2090	-.7283			43.96***	13.49***		
	TC	-.0381	-.8492				3.79		
	PC	.0622	-.9180			9.53***	7.27*		
	RTC	.2094	.0033	-.7306			.57	15.80***	4.86*
	RPC	.4302	.3076	-.7619			.39	27.76***	2.15
	TPC	-.1321	.1257	-.8546		.32	.		2.49
	RTPC	.5313	-.3218	.5194	-.5702	4.28	.26		.003
Consonant Errors PB	RC	.2013	-.6673			27.17**	7.82		
	TC	-.2785	-.6449				1.02		
	PC	.0971	-.8944			6.04	3.90		
	RTC	.1198	-.2541	-.5654		1.60	.21		9.29
	RPC	.4014	.2872	-.7037		.18	3.93	16.49***	1.23
	TPC	-.5282	.4265	-.7723			5.23*	.52	1.12
	RTPC	.5011	-.5856	.6998	-.5213	9.92*	.06		.69

time, contributes most to the multiple r, in terms of predictability. This is accomplished by testing the significance of the differences between the β weights. Tables 49 and 51 present results pertinent to this analysis. When predicting PB intelligibility from combinations of the variables, consonant errors, rhythm, time and phrases, all combinations including two, three and four predictor values are not appreciably higher than the value of .96 for PB consonant errors and PB intelligibility. Examination of the table further reveals that the only β weights significantly different from zero are for the consonant error predictor, when used in different combinations. The slight differences in predictable variance obtained when employing multiple correlation are probably not significant.

TABLE 51--Continued

Direction $F_{\beta_2-\beta_3}$	Absolute $F\|\beta_2\|-\|\beta_3\|$	Direction $F_{\beta_1-\beta_4}$	Absolute $F\|\beta_1\|-\|\beta_4\|$	Direction $F_{\beta_2-\beta_4}$	Absolute $F\|\beta_2\|-\|\beta_4\|$	Direction $F_{\beta_3-\beta_4}$	Absolute $F\|\beta_3\|-\|\beta_4\|$
	.01						
4.98* 1.94 1.65 4.02	1.87	24.60**	8.38*	9.19*	.84		2.04
15.53** 1.04	15.49** 11.78** 9.88** .13	42.83**	26.82**	16.83**	10.98**		9.42*
9.59*							
3.03** 12.47** 8.92* 3.10	2.98 2.25 4.93* .17	23.54**	.03		.30	14.30**	.03
.62 11.22** 10.07**	.06 6.32* .93 .08	22.86**	.02		.04	14.82**	.32

df = 1 & (N-n-1)

n = Number of predictors
N = Number in sample

		** $F_{.01}$	* $F_{.05}$
2 Predictors	F_{1-12}	9.33	4.75
3 Predictors	F_{1-11}	9.65	4.84
4 Predictors	F_{1-10}	10.04	4.96

F derived from Formula 12.50 and 12.51 in Truman Lee Kelley, Fundamentals of Statistics. Cambridge, Massachusetts: Harvard University Press, 1947, p. 478.

With respect to predicting sentence intelligibility from combinations of the variables, consonant errors, rhythm, time and phrases, none of the two predictor one criterion relationships offers any appreciably greater predictive information. The combination of rhythm, phrases and consonants offers an increase of 6 per cent greater predictive value than the 77 per cent predictable variance obtained for consonant errors and sentence intelligibility. When the four and five predictor one criterion relationships are considered, they offer an 8 per cent increase in predictable variance. For all combinations which include consonant errors as a variable the only β weight significantly different from zero is the β weight for the consonant errors. Table 49 further reveals that one combination, rhythm, time and phrases with sentence intelligibility offers the highest correlation when consonant errors are not considered. Furthermore, the β weights for each variable proved to be significantly different from zero. This suggests an analysis to determine which variable in this combination contributes most to the multiple r in terms of predictability. A consideration of the differences between the β's for this combination appears appropriate. Table 51 reveals that β_1 for rhythm is .86, and β_2 for time is —.74. The difference between the absolute numerical amount of .12 that each is contributing is not significant, but the algebraic difference of 1.6 is significant beyond the .01 level of confidence, indicating that these variables contribute approximately equal amounts in different directions. β_1, .86, rhythm; and β_3, .75, phrases, are both positive and the difference of .11 is not significant. They contribute approximately equal amounts in the same direction. β_2, —.74, time; and β_3, .75, phrases, contribute approximately equal amounts in opposite directions. Therefore, no conclusive statement can be made as to the variable which contributes most to the percentage of predictable variance.

REPORT OF SURGICAL DATA

Analysis of the data for the laryngectomized group as a whole and for the group classified according to high and low intelligibility (Table 54 in the Appendix) reveals no differentiating tendencies for the following factors investigated:

1. deep X-ray therapy previous to or following surgery,
2. radical neck dissection,
3. whether or not the epiglottis was removed with the larynx,
4. whether or not the strap muscles were removed with the larynx,
5. whether or not any of the esophagus was resected,

6. whether or not patient developed a fistula post-operatively.

For many surgeons, it is standard surgical procedure to remove as much of the tissue and muscle as necessary to prevent spread or recurrence of the malignancy. For the sample in this study the amount of tissue removed does not appear to have predictive value for intelligibility of speech.[1]

HISTORY INFORMATION

A portion of the history information (questions requesting the affirmative or negative reply) is summarized in Table 55 in the Appendix.

In regard to various questions raised in the literature the following trends were observed. Twelve of the fifteen subjects reported pre-operative hoarseness, and ten, coughing and loss of voice pre-operatively. Nine of the subjects indicated no apparent loss of ability to lift relatively heavy weights; fourteen, post-operative impairment of olfactory sensations; eight, impairment of gustatory sensations. The majority suggested improvement with time for both sensations. Eight reported increased fatigue and discomfort since the operation. None of the individuals had received speech training prior to surgery. Nine reported ability to "belch or burp" voluntarily before the operation (six of these individuals were judged to be low in intelligibility). Writing was usually employed immediately after surgery, and the length of training before engaging in conversation was highly variable, ranging from one month to six years. The majority indicated difficulty in talking in "noisy" situations, when under tension, after and during meals, and when lying down. Considerable satisfaction was derived from visits from another laryngectomized individual before and after surgery. There was little or no reported change in pre- and post-operative leisure time activities. No evident trends were observable when the questionnaire data were classified according to intelligibility groupings.

---

[1] A recent study by Dr. Evelyn M. Yellow Robe, *A Study of the Role of Three Factors in the Development of Speech After Laryngectomy: Type of Operation, Site of Pseudoglottis, and Coordination of Speech with Respiration.* Chicago: Northwestern University, 1954. Pp. 241. Mic A 54-2737; indicated that the type of laryngectomy for her sample did not appear significant in the success or failure of her group to develop voice production.

TENTATIVE CONCLUSIONS BASED ON THE ANALYSIS OF THE CINEFLUOROGRAPHIC FILM VIEWS

Drs. Irl Blaisdell and David Brewer, cooperating laryngologists, furnished the interpretations for the cinefluoroscopic phenomena. They reported the following trends:

1. The five laryngectomized speakers (high in intelligibility) did not appear to employ swallowing behavior, but instead the intake of air was limited to the proximal portion of the esophagus. For the five laryngectomized speakers judged to be low in intelligibility the film views illustrated decided swallowing behavior which propelled the air into the medial or lower two-thirds of the esophagus with some escape into the stomach.

2. The site of the pseudo-glottis for the laryngectomized speakers (high in intelligibility) appeared to be a small narrow vibrating portion of the esophagus in the approximate region of the reconstructed crico-pharyngeal sphincter. For the laryngectomized speakers (low in intelligibility) the pseudo-glottis occupied a relatively larger vibrating portion extending below the reconstructed crico-pharyngeal sphincter.

3. The film also provided a partial answer to the question of the relationship of amplitude measurements (excursion of the body walls) and the site of the pseudo-glottis. The film revealed greater abdominal movement for the poorer speakers. The kymograph amplitude measurements and the film information for the limited sample in this portion of the study substantiated the hypothesis offered by the medical profession, and substantiated by Anderson, that the lower the pseudo-glottis, the greater the abdominal amplitude, and the higher the pseudo-glottis, the greater the thoracic amplitude (excursion of the chest walls).

4. The laryngectomized speakers with high intelligibility were able to complete the passage in the exposure period; while the poorer speakers did not complete the passage in the same period of time. This finding is consistent with the kymograph results in this study.

5. The film also indicates that the speech coordinations of the better speakers more closely approximated those of the normal speaker in the film. This supports one of the essential hypotheses of the study.

CHAPTER FIVE

SUMMARY AND CONCLUSIONS

THIS STUDY WAS DESIGNED TO COMPARE THE BREATH-ing and speech coordinations of fifteen normal and fifteen laryngec-tomized speakers. Furthermore, the articulation and rhythm adequacy of the laryngectomized individuals was related to their intelligibility and speech coordinations.

The following hypotheses were examined:

1. That the speech coordinations of the laryngectomized would approximate those of the normal speaker.
2. That the quantitative intelligibility indexes employed in this study would differentiate between the better and poorer laryngec-tomized speakers.
3. That laryngectomized speakers who would be judged to be most intelligible would continue to employ breathing and speech coordinations more like the normal than do those who would be judged to be less intelligible.

Finally the investigation purported to gain an understanding of some of the predictive variables of intelligibility from the laryngectomized speakers.

A. Subjects
1. Fifteen adult laryngectomized individuals all employing speech accompanied by phonation for communication without use of artificial larynx.
2. Group of fifteen normal-speaking adults. The laryngectomized and the normal groups were matched for mean age and age range.

B. Instrumentation
1. A pneumatic method of recording was used throughout the experiment, employing a motor-driven variable speed kymo-graph.
2. Tape recordings of speech materials were made for each laryn-gectomized speaker.

C. Materials
1. Written material was read orally by the normal and laryngec-tomized speakers and comprised the following:

    a. six groups of four syllables each and one group of eight syllables each,

    b. a five-syllable phrase,

    c. a seven-syllable phrase,

    d. a nine-syllable phrase,

    e. a sixty-syllable paragraph.

D. Procedures

The following kymograph records were secured for the fifteen normal and fifteen laryngectomized subjects. The records were made under conditions of silent breathing and under oral reading conditions.

1. Silent breathing records; tracing of the movements of the body wall at the lower sternum area and mesogastric area.

2. Breathing for speech records.

    a. tracing of the movements of the body wall at the lower sternum area and the mesogastric area,

    b. tracing of the syllable pulse,

    c. tracing of the air pressure inside of the mouth, outside of the mouth and a combined inside and outside measurement.

E. Measurements and analysis

1. Silent breathing.

    a. Silent breathing records were measured for the amplitude of the breathing curves.

    b. The number of breathing cycles per minute were determined.

2. Speech breathing.

The sixty-syllable paragraph records were measured for:

    a. the total time in speaking the paragraph,

    b. the number of phrases employed in speaking the paragraph,

    c. the abdominal, chest and combined amplitude measured in millimeters for the phrasing movements.

Records of the five-, seven- and nine-syllable phrases were measured for:

    a. total time in speaking the phrases,

    b. number of phrases employed in speaking,

    c. the abdominal, chest and combined amplitude measured in millimeters for the phrasing movements.

Comparisons of configuration patterns for the tracings of the air pressure inside the mouth, outside the mouth and a combined inside and outside measurement where made.

    F. Judged intelligibility of the laryngectomized subjects
        1. Materials.
           a. fifty monosyllabic words (PB),
           b. Haagen's Multiple Choice Intelligibility Test, consisting of eight three-word phrases,
           c. ten sentences varying in the number of syllables.

Each speaker read different material in each of the categories mentioned above. All material was recorded under standardized conditions on tape.

        2. Auditors.
           a. A group of speech pathology and audiology majors served as auditors for the intelligibility portion of the study. The initial auditing group consisted of speech pathology and audiology majors and non-speech pathology and audiology majors. Statistical treatment of the auditing scores indicated a significant difference between the two groups, and the scores could not be combined.
           b. The speech pathology and audiology majors' auditing scores were selected as providing the most optimal listening conditions.
        3. Intelligibility scores.
           a. Standardized scoring formulas and audition recording forms were employed.
           b. Each speaker was given a separate percentage intelligibility score for the sentences, the fifty PB words, and for Haagen's multiple choice test.
           c. The use of standard scores permitted the computation of a combined standard score for the three intelligibility tests.
        4. Phonetic and error analysis of PB and sentence material was completed for the laryngectomized speakers. Two types of error analyses were employed:
           a. sound categories,
           b. types of errors.
        5. A rhythm analysis of the 150 sentences spoken by the laryngectomized speakers was undertaken.
        6. Surgical and history information was secured.
        7. A cinefluorographic film of the physiological and anatomical

mechanism involved in speech after laryngectomy was made of ten laryngectomized speakers and one normal speaker.

8. Statistical analysis was completed of the differences found between the breathing and speech coordinations of the laryngectomized and the normal speakers.

9. The speech coordinations, articulation and rhythm factors for the laryngectomized speakers were related to their intelligibility.

10. Further analysis was made between the normal group and laryngectomized speakers judged to be high in intelligibility with those judged to be low in intelligibility.

CONCLUSIONS

This study permits the following tentative conclusions for the sample employed.

1. The laryngectomized speakers differ significantly from the normal group in silent breathing, exhibiting a greater number of breathing cycles per minute and having greater chest amplitude. Although these differences in silent breathing are statistically significant, they are not considered to have critical clinical importance. The kymograph tracings for the normal and laryngectomized speakers reveal marked similarity in configuration.

2. The laryngectomized speakers in this study differ significantly from the normal group in speech breathing with particular differences revealed in the total time and the number of phrases employed in speaking the five-, seven- and nine-syllable phrases and the sixty-syllable paragraph. Laryngectomized speakers use greater time and more phrases. Chest and abdominal amplitude measurements for the sixty-syllable paragraph do not reveal significant differences between the groups.

3. The intelligibility indexes: (a) sentences, (b) phonetically balanced words and (c) the multiple choice test, differentiate between the laryngectomized speakers on the basis of intelligibility.

4. Those laryngectomized speakers who are judged to be most intelligible approached the speech coordinations of the normal subjects more closely than those laryngectomized speakers who are judged to be less intelligible. The kymograph tracings and the distribution of variable scores (time and phrases) substantiate this fact.

5. Articulatory analysis of sound error categories reveals a proportionally similar distribution between the consonant and vowel errors.

6. The sound categories listed from most to least intelligible according to the percentages of the sounds in the various categories produced correctly are:
   a. Glides,
   b. Laterals,
   c. Stop plosives,
   d. Final consonants,
   e. Vowels,
   f. Voiceless consonants
   g. Voiced consonants,
   h. Initial consonants,
   i. Fricatives,
   j. Nasals.

7. Articulatory analysis of consonant error types indicate that the releasing and arresting consonants present the greater percentage of errors for the sentences than for PB material. No significant differences exist for the remaining consonant error types for these materials.

8. For the sentence material, the surd-sonant, releasing and arresting consonant errors are significantly related to sentence intelligibility. Substitution and vowel errors are also significantly related to sentence intelligibility.

9. For the PB material, every consonant error category, with the exception of the releasing consonant errors, is significantly related to PB intelligibility. Substitution and neutralization vowel errors also relate significantly to intelligibility.

10. For both sound error categories and error types, the low intelligibility laryngectomized speakers persist in producing greater percentages of errors.

11. The predictors of intelligibility which contribute the greatest percentage of predictable variance prove to be consonant errors, rhythm, time and phrases respectively. Consonant errors for both PB and sentence material provide the highest correlations and greatest percentage of predictable variance when related to intelligibility. This relationship persists for all multiple correlations.

Examination of the configurations of the kymograph tracings and cinefluorographic film views in conjunction with the intelligibility scores reveals synchrony of the inspiratory and expiratory phases of respiration in gross and small detail for the laryngectomized speakers high in intelligibility. For the laryngectomized speakers judged to be low in intelligibility, the tracings definitely indicate dysynchrony of the inspiration-expiration phases in both gross and small detail. The findings of this study indicate a tendency toward synchronization of intake of air in the mouth and the inspiratory phases of the abdomen and thorax (Figures 17, 18, 19, 20 and 23).[1] The laryngectomized speakers with low intelligibility scores manifest speech breathing coordinations which tend to break down and reduce the efficiency of the respiration-phonation process. The data and analysis in this study substantially support Stetson, Burger and Kaiser's observations and findings that laryngectomized individuals continue to use normal speech coordinations in the speech relearning process.

The laryngectomized speaker should learn to utilize the air supply to coincide with normal speech coordinations most efficiently, through proper intake and control of the air column for voice production. It would appear desirable to develop synchronous speech-breathing co-ordinations and voice control prior to the development of communicative speech. The process would emphasize "relaxation" techniques which would help develop more adequate control of the air column and voice production. During this process after adequate prolongation of voice has been established, the voice should be fused with articulatory movements into proper feet and accent patterns.

This type of approach would help to establish rhythm and phrasing units prior to communicative speech. Under such conditions respiration and phonation would be closely associated, and the entire process could be formulated within the framework of an adequate learning theory in which success with voice control would represent goal attainment and primary reinforcement. Primary and secondary reinforcement would facilitate extension to the articulatory process. These results should culminate in a more satisfactory communication instruction situation whereby the mechanics of speech retraining would develop on a level of unawareness and would circumvent the acquisition of extraneous and unnecessary muscular behavior, which would provide distraction and enhance unintelligibility.

APPENDIX

TABLE 52

TABLE 52

IDENTIFYING INFORMATION OF NORMAL SPEAKERS INDICATING
MEAN AND MEDIAN AGES AND AGE RANGE

Number	Name	Age
1	A.P.	74
2	W.P.	67
3	P.H.S.	61
4	A.L.	54
5	T.B.	50
6	H.G.	59
7	E.M.	37
8	G.H.	57
9	D.C.	54
10	G.M.	68
11	J.I.	68
12	M.G.	58
13	A.O.	69
14	F.H.B.	57
15	T.M.	68

$\overline{X}$ Age = 60.1
Median Age = 59.0   Age Range 37 - 70

TABLE 53

IDENTIFYING INFORMATION OF LARYNGECTOMIZED SPEAKERS
ACCORDING TO INTELLIGIBILITY GROUPS INDICATING
MEAN AND MEDIAN AGES AND AGE RANGE

Number	Name	Age	Intelligibility Group		Pre-operative Occupation	Present Occupation	Time Interval Between Surgery and Experiment
			+z̄ N = 7	-z̄ N = 8			
1	P.S.	61	X		Salesman	Retired	5 1/2 years
2	M.G.	55	X		Contractor	Contractor	3 years
3	S.L.	61	X		Accountant	Accountant	2 1/2 years
4	L.J.	61	X		Salesman	Salesman	1 year
5	C.M.	74		X	Woodworker	Retired	2 1/2 years
6	O.R.	70		X	Telegrapher	Retired	1 year
7	J.K.	67		X	Machinist	Retired	8 years
8	C.K.	58		X	Painter	Unemployed	2 years
9	F.F.	69		X	Stock Clerk	Stock Clerk	4 1/2 years
10	P.L.M.	55		X	Barber	Barber	3 years
11	H.G.	36	X		Business Executive	Business Executive	6 months
12	F.M.	64	X		Salesman	Sales Supervisor	5 1/2 years
13	H.V.	49	X		Factory Supervisor	Factory Supervisor	1 1/2 years
14	G.B.	60		X	School Superintendent	Retired	2 years
15	M.A.	58		X	Merchant	Merchant	3 years

X̄ Age = 59.9
Median Age = 60.8   Age Range = 36 - 74

TABLE 54

SURGICAL DATA DIVIDED ACCORDING TO
INTELLIGIBILITY GROUPS

Surgical Data	+z̄ Group N = 7		-z̄ Group N = 8	
	Yes	No	Yes	No
Deep X-ray therapy previous to or following surgery	1	6	0	8
Radical neck dissection	2	5	0	8
Removal of epiglottis	6	1	7	1
Removal of strap muscles	5	2	7	1
Resection of any portion of esophagus	1	6	1	7
Post-operative fistula	2	5	5	3

TABLE 55

PARTIAL SUMMARY OF HISTORY INFORMATION

N = 15	Item	+z̄ Group High Intelligibility N = 7		−z̄ Group Low Intelligibility N = 8	
		Yes	No	Yes	No
1.	Speech training prior to surgery	0	7	0	8
2.	Ability to belch before operation	3	4	6	2
3.	Ability to produce audible speech	6	1	8	0
4.	Ability to produce intelligible speech	3	4	5	3
5.	Difficulty speaking when frightened	6	1	4	4
6.	Difficulty speaking when angry	1	6	5	3
7.	Confidence in ability to instruct another laryngectomized individual	6	1	3	5
8.	Experience in instructing others to speak	4	3	1	7
9.	Pre-operative visit by laryngectomized speaker . .	3	4	5	3
10.	Experience in visiting laryngectomized individuals	6	1	2	6
11.	Smoking at present	2	5	5	3
12.	Smoking prior to operation	6	1	8	0
13.	Ability to lift heavy weights	4	3	5	3
14.	Post-operative change in the ability to lift heavy weights	3	4	5	3
15.	Pre-operative hoarseness	6	1	6	2
16.	Pre-operative pain	2	5	0	8
17.	Pre-operative coughing	6	1	4	4
18.	Pre-operative loss of voice	5	2	5	3
19.	Post-operative impairment of olfactory sensation .	7	0	7	1
20.	Post-operative impairment of gustatory sensation .	5	2	3	5
21.	Ability to sneeze at present	7	0	7	1
22.	Change in breathing ability associated with changes in weather	5	2	3	5
23.	Change in speaking ability associated with changes in weather	5	2	1	7
24.	Increased fatigue since operation	2	5	6	2
25.	Increased discomfort since operation	3	4	5	3

TABLE 56

REPEATED MEASUREMENTS ON THE SAME KYMOGRAPH TRACINGS FOR NORMAL AND LARYNGECTOMIZED SPEAKERS IN SILENT AND SPEECH BREATHING BY FIVE READERS AND FOR FIVE SERIES OF MEASURES BY THE EXPERIMENTER IN MILLIMETERS INDICATING MEANS FOR EACH SUB-GROUP AND TOTALS

Measure		Consistency of Five Individuals Making Fifty Measurements					Consistency of the Experimenter Making Fifty Measurements					Number of Measurements
		A	B	C	D	E	1	2	3	4	5	
Normal Speakers — Silent Breathing		13.0	13.0	13.0	13.0	13.0	13.0	13.0	13.0	13.0	13.0	
		11.5	11.0	11.5	11.0	11.0	11.0	11.0	11.0	11.0	11.5	
		11.0	11.0	11.0	10.5	11.0	11.0	11.0	11.0	11.0	11.0	
		11.0	11.0	11.0	11.0	11.0	11.0	11.0	11.0	11.0	11.0	
		12.5	12.0	12.0	12.0	12.0	12.0	12.0	12.0	12.0	12.0	
		13.0	13.0	13.0	13.0	13.0	13.0	13.0	12.5	12.5	12.5	
		12.0	11.5	12.0	11.5	11.5	11.5	11.5	11.5	11.5	11.5	
		11.0	11.0	11.0	11.0	11.0	11.0	11.0	11.0	11.0	11.0	
		11.0	11.0	11.0	11.0	11.0	10.5	10.5	11.0	11.0	10.5	
		13.0	12.5	13.0	13.0	13.0	12.5	12.5	12.5	12.5	12.5	
Normal Speakers — Speech Breathing		11.0	11.0	11.0	11.0	11.0	11.0	11.0	11.0	11.0	11.0	
		20.0	19.5	19.5	19.5	19.5	19.5	19.0	19.5	19.0	19.5	
		18.0	18.0	18.0	18.0	18.0	18.0	18.0	18.0	18.0	18.0	
		6.0	6.0	6.0	6.0	6.0	6.0	6.0	6.0	6.0	6.0	
		12.0	11.5	12.0	12.0	11.5	11.5	11.5	11.5	11.5	11.5	
		16.0	15.5	15.5	15.5	15.5	15.5	15.5	15.0	15.5	15.5	
		13.0	13.0	13.0	13.0	13.0	13.0	13.0	13.0	13.0	13.0	
		2.0	2.0	2.0	2.0	2.0	2.0	2.0	2.0	2.0	2.0	
		16.5	16.5	16.5	16.5	16.0	16.5	16.0	16.0	16.0	16.0	
		8.0	8.0	8.0	8.0	8.0	8.0	8.0	8.0	8.0	8.0	
		10.0	10.0	10.0	10.0	10.0	10.0	10.0	10.0	10.0	10.0	
		7.0	7.0	7.0	7.0	7.0	7.0	7.0	7.0	7.0	7.0	
		12.0	12.0	12.5	12.5	12.0	12.0	12.0	12.0	12.0	12.0	
Laryngectomized Speakers — Silent Breathing		22.0	22.0	22.0	22.0	22.5	22.0	22.0	22.0	22.0	22.0	
		17.0	17.0	17.0	17.0	17.0	17.0	17.0	17.0	17.0	17.0	
		17.0	17.0	17.0	17.0	17.0	17.0	17.0	17.0	17.0	17.0	
		13.0	13.0	13.0	13.0	13.5	13.0	13.0	13.0	13.0	13.5	
		15.0	15.0	15.0	15.0	15.0	15.0	15.0	15.0	15.0	15.0	
		6.5	6.0	6.5	6.5	7.0	6.5	6.5	6.5	6.5	7.0	
		21.0	20.5	20.5	21.0	21.0	21.0	21.0	21.0	21.0	21.0	
		12.5	12.0	12.5	12.5	12.5	12.5	12.5	12.5	12.0	12.5	
		4.0	4.0	4.0	4.0	4.0	4.0	4.0	4.0	4.0	4.0	
		6.5	6.5	6.0	6.5	6.5	6.5	6.5	6.5	6.5	6.5	
Laryngectomized Speakers — Speech Breathing		20.0	20.0	20.0	20.0	20.0	20.0	20.0	20.0	20.0	20.0	
		22.0	22.0	22.0	22.0	22.0	22.0	22.0	22.0	22.0	22.0	
		6.0	6.5	6.0	6.5	6.5	6.0	6.5	6.5	6.5	6.0	
		15.5	15.0	15.0	15.5	15.5	15.5	15.5	15.5	15.5	15.5	
		4.0	4.0	4.0	4.0	4.0	4.0	4.0	4.0	4.0	4.0	
		10.0	10.0	10.0	10.0	10.0	10.0	10.0	10.0	10.0	10.0	
		18.5	18.5	18.5	18.5	19.0	18.5	18.5	18.5	18.5	18.5	
		7.0	7.5	7.0	7.5	8.0	7.0	7.5	7.0	7.5	7.0	
		11.5	11.0	11.0	11.0	11.0	11.5	11.5	11.0	11.5	11.5	
		5.0	5.0	5.0	5.0	5.5	5.0	5.0	5.0	5.0	5.0	
		8.0	8.0	8.0	8.0	8.0	8.0	8.0	8.0	8.0	8.0	
		6.5	6.5	7.0	6.5	6.5	6.5	6.5	6.5	6.5	7.0	
		5.5	5.5	5.5	5.5	6.0	5.5	5.5	5.5	5.5	5.5	
		3.0	3.0	3.0	3.0	3.0	3.0	3.0	3.0	3.0	3.0	
		6.0	6.0	6.0	6.0	6.0	6.0	6.0	6.0	6.0	6.0	
Normal	Silence $\bar{X}$	11.90	11.70	11.85	11.70	11.75	11.65	11.65	11.65	11.65	11.65	10
	Speech $\bar{X}$	10.70	10.60	10.70	10.67	10.57	10.57	10.50	10.50	10.50	10.53	15
Laryngec- tomized	Silence $\bar{X}$	13.45	13.30	13.35	13.45	13.60	13.45	13.45	13.45	13.40	13.55	10
	Speech $\bar{X}$	9.90	9.90	9.87	9.93	10.07	9.90	9.97	9.90	9.97	9.93	15
Total	$\bar{X}$	11.25	11.15	11.21	11.21	11.26	11.16	11.16	11.14	11.15	11.01	50

Correlation coefficients:
Individuals A and B = .9989
C and D = .9992

Experimenter measurements
2 and 5 = .9992

TABLE 57

RELATIVE FREQUENCY OF CONSONANTS IN SENTENCE TEST MATERIALS OF
PRESENT STUDY AND IN DEWEY'S ANALYSIS OF TEN THOUSAND
WORDS IN TESTS OF PERCENTAGE OF TOTAL SOUNDS

Sound	Frequency	
	Present Study	Dewey's Study
[r]	8.05	6.88
[t]	7.70	7.13
[n]	6.82	7.24
[ð]	6.55	3.43
[d]	4.76	4.31
[s]	4.48	4.55
[l]	4.20	3.74
[k]	3.65	2.71
[z]	3.13	2.97
[w]	2.94	2.08
[h]	2.90	1.81
[p]	2.54	2.04
[b]	2.42	1.81
[m]	2.14	2.78
[f]	1.55	1.84
[v]	1.27	2.28
[tʃ]	1.07	.52
[ʃ]	1.03	.82
[ŋ]	.99	.96
[dʒ]	.75	.44
[g]	.48	.74
[θ]	.32	.37
[j]	.24	.60
[ʍ]	.16	*
[ʒ]	.08	.05

*Not included in Dewey's list.

Sample of the Three Types of Material Utilized for Judging the Speech Intelligibility of the Laryngectomized Speakers
(*Speaker P.L.M.*)

Materials Recorded on Magnecorder

PB-50 LIST 16 (RANDOMIZED)

1. Rock	11. Map	21. Louse	31. Aid	41. Book
2. Next	12. Barge	22. Pump	32. Wield	42. Gas
3. Cheese	13. Lay	23. Turn	33. Soar	43. Rug
4. Knee	14. Crews	24. Thou	34. Gab	44. Nap
5. Dame	15. Rye	25. Sang	35. Stab	45. Suit
6. Rogue	16. Pitch	26. Hash	36. Droop	46. Fright
7. Stress	17. Kind	27. Sheep	37. Tuck	47. Ink
8. Hose	18. Tire	28. Three	38. Leash	48. Ton
9. Sheik	19. Had	29. Dub	39. Fifth	49. Cliff
10. Closed	20. Drape	30. Thresh	40. Part	50. Din

HAAGEN MULTIPLE CHOICE TEST NO. 14

1. Muzzle, Carve, Author
2. Scorch, Able, Cloth
3. Vision, Fumble, Grown
4. Cape, Lecture, High
5. Possess, Blow, Single
6. Divide, Fiction, Maker
7. Leaf, Section, Rich
8. Traitor, Eastward, Join

LIST OF TEN SENTENCES

1. The radio was turned on. 2. The clock struck twelve. 3. Spring is a delightful time of year. 4. The tomato juice was chilled. 5. He bought a new pair of shoes. 6. The hurricane roared with great fury. 7. The band played a marching song. 8. He placed the black brief case on the table. 9. The stars were bright last night. 10. Are you going home tomorrow?

Research in Speech After Laryngectomy

GORDON D. HOOPLE HEARING AND SPEECH CENTER
Syracuse University
805 South Crouse Avenue
Syracuse, New York

SURGICAL REPORT

Name_____ Age_____ Address_____

I. Did the patient have any deep X-ray therapy previous to or following surgery?

   _____
   _____

II. Was a radical neck dissection also done?_____

   _____

III. Was the epiglottis removed with the larynx?_____

   _____

IV. Were the strap muscles removed with the larynx?_____

   _____

V. Was any of the esophagus resected?_____

   _____

VI. Did the patient develop a fistula post operatively?_____

   _____

Date of Surgery _____

Hospital _____ Address_____

Surgeon _____

Date of report_____

Research in Speech After Laryngectomy

GORDON D. HOOPLE HEARING AND SPEECH CENTER
805 South Crouse Avenue
Syracuse, New York

HISTORY INFORMATION

Name _____ Age_____ Date of Birth_____

Address _____ Single_____ Married_____

Telephone _____ Children_____ Ages _____

Present Occupation _____ Dates of Surgery_____

Retired _____ Name of Surgeon_____

Education: Grammar School _____ Hospital _____

          High School _____ Address _____

          College _____

Instructions: Please circle a yes or no answer; indicate with a check
mark where it is required; and where specific information
is called for, please give the necessary details. If further
space is required, please use reverse side of sheets.

1. Did you receive any training in learning to speak prior to your
operation? YES, NO. If the answer is yes, please describe._____

2. Were you able to voluntarily belch before the operation? YES,
NO.

3. How did you communicate immediately after the operation, before
you learned to speak? *Please Check* (a) Artificial larynx_____,
(b) Whispered speech_____, (c) Writing_____, (d) Gestures.
How long did you use such methods?_____

4. How soon after surgery did you make an attempt to learn to speak?

5. Who taught you to speak? (a) Self taught. YES, NO. If self
taught, did you read any material on the subject? YES, NO.
What material? _____

(b) Taught by others.
     1) Physician. YES, NO. Total number hours of therapy.
        _____ Individual therapy? _____ Group therapy?
        _____

    2) Laryngectomized individual? YES, NO. Total number of hours of therapy._____ Individual therapy?_____ Group therapy? _____

    3) Speech Correctionist? YES, NO. Total number of hours of therapy. _____ Individual therapy? _____ Group therapy? _____

6. How soon after you began special training (either alone or with help) were you able to say your first sound? _____; your first word? _____; your first sentence? _____; engage in regular conversation?_____.

7. Are you usually able to make yourself heard when speaking? YES, NO. If not, please describe the situation in which you experience difficulty. _____

8. Do people indicate that they have not understood you? YES, NO. How often does this occur?_____
    (a) How do you handle these situations?_____
    _____
    (b) How do you react to these situations?_____
    _____

9. How often do people question you about your voice?_____
    (a) What comments do you make to such questioning?_____
    _____

10. How do you feel about talking to strangers?_____
    _____

11. Under what conditions do you speak best?_____
    _____

12. Under what conditions do you speak poorest?_____
    _____

13. Do you have difficulty speaking when you are frightened? YES, NO, or when you are angry? YES, NO. If so, please describe.___
    _____
    _____

14. In what position (or positions) is it easiest for you to speak? Standing _____ Sitting _____ Lying down _____ Please explain:
    _____
    _____

15. Do you feel able to teach a laryngectomized individual to speak? YES, NO.

16. Have you taught any laryngectomized individuals to speak? YES NO. Number of individuals?_____

17. If you were able to teach another laryngectomized person to speak, how would you explain your method to him?_____
   _____
   _____
   _____
   _____

18. Did a laryngectomized speaker visit you? YES, NO.
   (a) Before the operation? _____ (b) Shortly after the operation? _____ What was your reaction to these visits?_____
   _____

19. Have you visited any laryngectomized individuals? YES, NO.
   (a) Before the operation? _____ (b) After the operation? _____ What were your reactions to this situation?_____
   _____

20. What type of shirt do you wear?_____
   What type of collar?_____
   What type of tie?_____

21. Do you smoke now?_____
   _____
   How do you accomplish this?_____
   _____

22. Did you smoke before the operation? YES, NO. Pipe? _____
   Cigar? _____ Cigarettes? _____ Were you a heavy smoker?
   _____ Average? _____ Light? _____ Infrequent? _____

23. What was your occupation before the operation?_____
   _____

24. Can you lift heavy weights? YES, NO. Is there a difference in your ability to do this, since the operation? YES, NO. Please describe. _____
   _____

25. Prior to your operation, did you have any condition of hoarseness _____, pain _____ or coughing, or loss of voice? _____
   How long did any of these conditions last before you saw a throat specialist? _____

26. After the operation was your sense of smell affected? YES, NO. In what way?_____
   _____

27. After the operation was your sense of taste affected? YES, NO. In what way?_____

28. Has there been any change in these senses since then? YES, NO. Please describe. _____

29. Are you able to sneeze? YES, NO. If so, please explain how this is accomplished. _____

30. (a) Do changes in weather affect your breathing? YES, NO. Please describe. _____
    (b) Do changes in weather affect your speaking? YES, NO. Please describe. _____

31. Since the operation has any increased fatigue been noticed? YES, NO. Any increased discomfort? YES, NO. Please describe.____

32. Do you have frequent coughing spells? YES, NO. _____

33. Were you aware that you had a condition of cancer before the operation? YES, NO. _____

34. Did you know that you would be unable to speak after the operation? YES, NO.

35. (a) What clubs or organizations are you a member (or associated with) at the present time?_____
    (b) What clubs or organizations were you a member (or associated with) just prior to your illness?_____

36. (a) What leisure time recreational activities do you engage in at the present time?_____
    (b) What leisure time recreational activities did you engage in just prior to your illness?_____

37. Are you satisfied with your speech as it is now? Please explain. _____

Signature _____

Date _____

Auditor's Scoring Sheet for Haagen Multiple Choice Test

Auditor's Name_____ Intelligibility Score_____

Speaker's Name_____ Date_____

Speaker 10 is P.L.M.

1 puddle	1 carve	1 offer
2 muddle	2 car	2 author
3 muzzle	3 tarred	3 often
4 puzzle	4 tired	4 office
1 porch	1 fable	1 cross
2 torch	2 stable	2 cough
3 scorch	3 table	3 cloth
4 court	4 able	4 claw
1 vision	1 bubble	1 thrown
2 bishop	2 tumble	2 drone
3 vicious	3 stumble	3 prone
4 season	4 fumble	4 groan
1 cape	1 texture	1 eye
2 hate	2 lecture	2 high
3 take	3 mixture	3 tie
4 tape	4 rupture	4 hide
1 process	1 glow	1 single
2 protest	2 blow	2 jingle
3 profess	3 below	3 cycle
4 possess	4 low	4 sprinkle
1 divide	1 kitchen	1 baker
2 devise	2 mission	2 major
3 define	3 friction	3 maker
4 divine	4 fiction	4 banker
1 leap	1 second	1 rich
2 leaf	2 suction	2 ridge
3 lease	3 section	3 bridge
4 leave	4 sexton	4 grip
1 crater	1 seaport	1 joy
2 traitor	2 keyboard	2 going
3 trainer	3 piecework	3 join
4 treasure	4 eastward	4 dawn

Auditor's Recording Sheet for Sentence Test

Auditor's Name_____ Intelligibility Score_____

Speaker's Name_____ Date_____

  1. a. _____

       b. _____

       c. _____

  2. a. _____

       b. _____

       c. _____

  3. a. _____

       b. _____

       c. _____

  4. a. _____

       b. _____

       c. _____

  5. a. _____

       b. _____

       c. _____

  6. a. _____

       b. _____

       c. _____

  7. a. _____

       b. _____

       c. _____

  8. a. _____

       b. _____

       c. _____

  9. a. _____

       b. _____

       c. _____

10. a. _____

       b. _____

       c. _____

Auditor's Recording Sheet for PB Word List

Auditor's Name_____ Intelligibility Score_____

Speaker's Name_____ Date_____

1	_____	26 _____
2	_____	27 _____
3	_____	28 _____
4	_____	29 _____
5	_____	30 _____
6	_____	31 _____
7	_____	32 _____
8	_____	33 _____
9	_____	34 _____
10	_____	35 _____
11	_____	36 _____
12	_____	37 _____
13	_____	38 _____
14	_____	39 _____
15	_____	40 _____
16	_____	41 _____
17	_____	42 _____
18	_____	43 _____
19	_____	44 _____
20	_____	45 _____
21	_____	46 _____
22	_____	47 _____
23	_____	48 _____
24	_____	49 _____
25	_____	50 _____

BIBLIOGRAPHY

1. Anderson, John O. Dean. "Study of Some Factors Concerning Esophageal Speech." Unpublished Doctoral dissertation, Ohio State University, 1951. Pp. 124.

2. Baker, H. K., and McDonald E. "Rehabilitation of the Laryngectomized," *Crippled Child,* XXVIII (October, 1950), 10-11.

3. Bangs, Jack L. "Bibliography: Esophageal Speech," *Journal of Speech Disorders,* XII (September, 1947), 339-341.

4. Bangs, Jack L., Lierle, D. M., and Strother, C. R. "Speech After Laryngectomy," *Journal of Speech Disorder,* XI (September, 1946), 171-176.

5. Bateman, B. M., Dornhorst, A. C., and Leathart, M. B. "Oesophageal Speech," *British Medical Journal,* II (November 29, 1952), 1177-1178.

6. Billroth, T., cited by Gussenbauer, C. "Ueber die erste durch Th. Billroth am Menschen ausgeführte Kehlkopfsexstirpation und die Anwendung eines Künstlichen Kehlkopes," *Arch. f. klin. Chir* 17:343, 1874 in Kallen, L. A. "Vicarious Vocal Mechanisms," *Archives of Otolaryngology,* XX (July-December, 1934), 460-503.

7. Brighton, G. R., and Boone, W. H. "Roentgenographic Demonstration of Method of Speech in Cases of Complete Laryngectomy," *American Journal of Roentgenology and Radium Therapy,* XXXVIII (July-December, 1937), 571-583.

8. Burger, H., and Kaiser, L. "Speech Without a Larynx," *Acta Otolaryngologica,* VIII (1925), 90-116.

9. Cypreansen, Lucile E. "An Investigation of the Breathing and Speech Coordinations and the Speech Intelligibility of Normal Speaking Children and of Cerebral Palsied Children with Speech Defects." Unpublished Ph.D. dissertation, Department of Education, Syracuse University, 1953. Pp. 220.

10. Czermak, J. "Ueber die Sprache bei luftdichter Verschliessung des Kehlkops," *Sitzungsb. d. K. Akad. d. Wissensch. Math. naturw. Cl., Wien* 35:65, 1859. Cited by Kallen, L. A. "Vicarious Vocal Mechanisms," *Archives of Otolaryngology,* XX (July-December, 1934), 460-503.

11. Dewey, Godfrey. *Relative Frequency of English Speech Sounds.* Cambridge, Massachusetts: Harvard University Press, 1923. Pp. 148.

12. Dornhorst, A. C., and Leathart, G. L. "A Method of Assessing the Mechanical Properties of Lungs and Air-passages," *The Lancet,* II (July 19, 1952), 109-111.

13. Edwards, Allen L. *Experimental Design in Psychological Research.* New York: Rinehart & Company, 1946. Pp. 446.

14. Egan, James P. "Articulation Testing Methods," *The Laryngoscope,* LVIII (September, 1948) , 955-991.

15. Gatewood, E. T. "A New and Simple Procedure for Developing Esophageal Voice in the Laryngectomized Patient," *Virginia Medical Monthly,* LXXIII (May, 1946) , 206-209.

16. Gatewood, E. T. "A Simple and Practical Procedure for Developing Esophageal Voice in the Laryngectomized Patient," *Annals of Otology, Rhinology, and Laryngology,* LIV (1945) , 322-327.

17. Gatewood, E. T. "The Mechanism of Esophageal Voice Following Laryngectomy," *Virginia Medical Monthly,* LXXI (January, 1944) , 9-13.

18. Gray, W. G., and Wise, C. M. *The Bases of Speech* (revised) . New York: Harper & Brothers, 1946. Pp. 610.

19. Greene, J. S. "Speech Rehabilitation Following Laryngectomy," *American Journal of Nursing,* XLIX (March, 1949), 153-154.

20. Gutzman, Herman, Sr. "Stimme und Sprache Ohne Kehlkopf," Ztschr. Laryng., Rhin., Otol. 1:221, 1909 cited by W. W. Morrison "The Production of Voice and Speech Following Total Laryngectomy," Archives of Otolaryngology, XIV (October, 1931) 413-431.

21. Haagen, C. Hess. "Intelligibility Measurement: Techniques and Procedures Used by the Voice Communication Laboratory," *USRD Report* No. 3748, PB 12169, May, 1948.

22. Harvard PB Lists Nos. 13 and 15, cited by H. Davis. *Hearing and Deafness.* New York: Murray Hill Book Co., Inc., 1947. Pp. 475.

23. Hudgins, C. V. "A Comparative Study of the Speech Coordinations of Deaf and Normal Subjects," *Pedagogical Seminary and Journal of Genetic Psychology,* XLIV (March, 1934) , 3-48.

24. Hudgins, C. V. "A Method of Appraising the Speech of the Deaf," *The Volta Review,* LI (December, 1949) , 593-640.

25. Hudgins, C. V. "The Research Program in Speech at the Clarke School," *The Volta Review,* LIV (October, 1952) , 355-362.

26. Hudgins, C. V., and Di Carlo, Louis M. "An Experimental Study of Assimilation Between Abutting Consonants," *Journal of General Psychology,* XX (April, 1939) , 449-469.

27. Hudgins, C. V., and Numbers, F. C. "An Investigation of the Intelligibility of the Speech of the Deaf," *Genetic Psychology Monographs,* XXV (1942) , 289-392.

28. Hudgins, C. V., and Stetson, R. H. "A Unit for Kymograph Recording," *Science,* LXXVI (July 15, 1932) , 59-60.

29. Hyman, M. "An Experimental Study of the Relative Pressure, Duration, Intelligibility and Aesthetic Aspects of the Speech of Artificial Larynx, Esophageal, and Normal Speakers." Unpublished Ph.D. dissertation, Ohio State University, 1953. Pp. 129.

30. Jackson, C. L. "The Voice After Direct Laryngoscopic Operations, Laryngofissure and Laryngectomy," *Archives of Otolaryngology,* XXXI (January-June, 1940), 23-37.

31. Johnson, Palmer O. *Statistical Methods in Research*. New York: Prentice Hall, 1949. Pp. 377.

32. Kallen, L. A. "Vicarious Vocal Mechanisms," *Archives of Otolaryngology*, XX (July-December, 1934), 460-503.

33. Kelley, Truman Lee. *Fundamentals of Statistics*. Cambridge, Massachusetts: Harvard University Press, 1947. Pp. 755.

34. Levin, N. M. "Speech Rehabilitation After Total Removal of Larynx," *The Journal of the American Medical Association*, CXL (August 2, 1952), 1281-1286.

35. Levin, N. M. "Teaching the Laryngectomized Patient to Talk," *Archives of Otolaryngology*, XXXII (July-December, 1940), 299-314.

36. Lindquist, E. F. *Statistical Analysis in Educational Research*. Boston: Houghton Mifflin Co., 1940. Pp. 266.

37. Lindsay, J. R., Morgan, R. H.. and Wepman, J. M. "The Cricopharyngeus Muscle in Esophageal Speech," *Laryngoscope*, LIV (February, 1944), 55-65.

38. McCall, J. W. "Preliminary Voice Training for Laryngectomy," *Archives of Otolaryngology*, XXXVIII (July-December, 1943), 10-16.

39. McNemar, Quinn. *Psychological Statistics*. New York: John Wiley and Son, Inc., 1949. Pp. 338.

40. Morrison, W. W. "Physical Rehabilitation of the Laryngectomized Patient," *Archives of Otolaryngology*, XXXIV (July-December, 1941), 1101-1112.

41. Morrison, W. W. "The Production of Voice and Speech Following Total Laryngectomy," *Archives of Otolaryngology*, XIV (October, 1931), 413-431.

42. Negus, V. E. "Affections of the Cricopharyngeal Fold," *Laryngoscope*, XLVIII (December, 1938), 847-858.

43. Nelson, Charles R. *You Can Speak Again:* Post-Laryngectomy Speech. New York: Funk & Wagnalls, 1949. Pp. 95.

44. Ogura, J. H., and Bello, J. A. "Laryngectomy and Radical Neck Dissection for Carcinoma of the Larynx," *Laryngoscope*, LXII (January, 1952), 1-52.

45. Orton, H. B. "A Review of the Available Literature on the Larynx and Laryngeal Surgery," *Laryngoscope*, LVIII (March, 1948), 181-205.

46. Rawlings, C. G. "A Comparative Study of the Movements of the Breathing Muscles in Speech and Quiet Breathing of Deaf and Normal Subjects," *American Annals of the Deaf*, LXXX (March, 1933), 147-156; and LXXXI, No. 2, (March, 1936), 136-150.

47. Romonek, P. L. "Artificial and Pseudo-voice Following Complete Laryngectomy," *Nebraska State Medical Journal*, XVII (June, 1932), 238-243.

48. Schall, L. A. "Psychology of Laryngectomized Patients," *Archives of Otolaryngology*, XXVIII (October, 1938), 581-584.

49. Schilling, R., and Binder, H. "Experimental Phonetische Untersuchungen über die Stimme ohne Kehlkopf," *Archiv für Ohren,-Nasen-und Kehlkopfheilkunde*, CXIV-CXV (1925-1926), 236-270.

50. Scripture, E. W. "Speech Without Using the Larynx," *Journal of Physiology,* L (December, 1915-1916), 397-403.

51. Seeman, M. "Phoniatrische Bemerkungen zur Laryngektomie," *Archiv für Klinische Chirurgie,* CXL (1926), 285-298.

52. Snedecor, G. W. *Statistical Methods.* Ames, Iowa: Iowa State-College Press. 1946. Pp. 485.

53. Stern, Hugo. "Der Mechanismus der Sprech-und Stimmbildung bei Laryngektomierten und die derartigen Fällen Angewandte Uebungstherapie," in Denker and Kahler: *Handbuch der Hals-Nasen-u. Ohrenheilkunde,* Berlin: Julius Springer, V (1926), 494, cited by Morrison, W. W. "The Production of Voice and Speech Following Total Laryngectomy," *Archives of Otolaryngology,* XIV (October, 1931), 413-431.

54. Stern, Hugo. "Grundprizipien der Sprache und Stimmausbildung bei Laryngektomierten nebst einem neuen Beitrag zum Mechanismus der Sprache und Stimme derartig Operierter," *Wien. Klin. Wschnschr,* XXXIII (1920), 540, cited by Kallen, L. A. "Vicarious Vocal Mechanisms," *Archives of Otolaryngology,* XX (July-December, 1934) 460-503.

55. Stetson, R. H. "Esophageal Speech for any Laryngectomized Patient," *Archives of Otolaryngology,* XXVI (July-December, 1937), 132-142.

56. Stetson, R. H. *Motor Phonetics: A Study of Speech Movements in Action.* Amsterdam: North-Holland Publishing Co., 1951. Pp. 212.

57. Stetson, R. H. "Oesophageal Speech: Methods of Instruction After Laryngectomy," *Archives Néerlandaises de Phonétique Expérimentale,* XIII (1937), 95-110.

58. Stetson, R. H. "Speech Movements in Action," *Transactions of the American Laryngological Association,* LV (1933), 29-41.

59. Stetson, R. H., and Hudgins, C. V. "Functions of the Breathing Movements in the Mechanism of Speech," *Archives Néerlandaises de Phonétique Expérimentale,* V (1930), 1-30.

60. Stoerk, K. "Ueber Larynxextirpation," *Wien. Med. Wchnschr.* 37:1535, 1887, cited by Morrison, W. W. "The Production of Voice and Speech Following Total Laryngectomy," *Archives of Otolaryngology,* XIV (October, 1931), 413-431.

61. Templeton, F. E., and Kredel, R. A. "The Cricopharyngeal Sphincter— A Roentgenologic Study," *Laryngoscope,* LIII (January, 1943), 1-12.

62. Thomson, St. Clair (Sir). "The History of Cancer of the Larynx," *Journal of Laryngology and Otology,* LIV (February, 1939), 61-87.

63. Walker, Crayton. "The Intrinsic Intensity of Oral Phrases." Unpublished Master's thesis, Ohio State University. Pp. 48.

64. Watson, J. S., Jr., and Weinberg, S. A. "A 35-Millimeter Unit for Cinefluorography," *Radiology,* LI (November, 1948), 728-732.

65. Weinberg, S. S., Watson, J. S., Jr., and Ramsey, G. H. "X-ray Motion Picture Techniques Employed in Medical Diagnosis and Research," *Journal of the SMPTE,* LIX (October, 1952), 300-308.